Melatonin - Recent Updates

Edited by Volkan Gelen, Emin Şengül and Abdulsamed Kükürt

Published in London, United Kingdom

Melatonin - Recent Updates
http://dx.doi.org/10.5772/intechopen.100989
Edited by Volkan Gelen, Emin Şengül and Abdulsamed Kükürt

Contributors
Mohammed Albreiki, Alicia González-González, Aurora Laborda-Illanes, Soukaina Boutriq, Lidia Sánchez-Alcoholado, Daniel Castellano-Castillo, Isaac Plaza-Andrades, Jesús Peralta-Linero, María Isabel Queipo Ortuño, Zekeriya Safa İnanç, Huzur Derya Arık, Oğuzhan Kahraman, Mustafa Selçuk Alataş, Adem Kara, Hülya Kara, Maria Rosa Avila Costa, Ana Luisa Gutiérrez-Valdez, Mariana Stephania Rodríguez-Alcántara, José Luis Ordóñez-Librado, Javier Sanchez-Betancourt, Enrique Montiel-Flores, Cesar Alfonso Garcia Caballero, Claudia Dorado-Martínez, Leonardo Reynoso-Erazo, Vianey Rodríguez-Lara, Jesús Espinosa-Villanueva, Patricia Aley-Medina, Rocío Tron-Alvarez, Volkan Gelen, Emin Şengül, Abdulsamed Kükürt, Oguz Merhan

First published in London, United Kingdom, 2022 by IntechOpen
IntechOpen is the global imprint of INTECHOPEN LIMITED, registered in England and Wales, registration number: 11086078, 5 Princes Gate Court, London, SW7 2QJ, United Kingdom

British Library Cataloguing-in-Publication Data
A catalogue record for this book is available from the British Library

Additional hard and PDF copies can be obtained from orders@intechopen.com

Melatonin - Recent Updates
Edited by Volkan Gelen, Emin Şengül and Abdulsamed Kükürt
p. cm.
Print ISBN 978-1-80356-734-1
Online ISBN 978-1-80356-735-8
eBook (PDF) ISBN 978-1-80356-736-5

Meet the editors

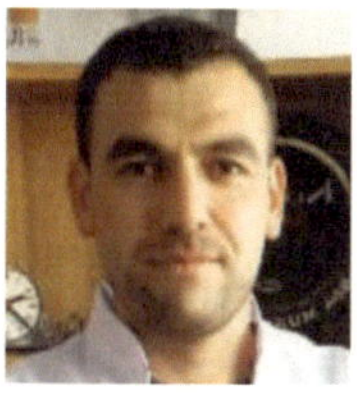

Dr. Volkan Gelen is a physiology specialist who received his veterinary degree from Kafkas University, Turkey, in 2011. From 2011 to 2015, he worked as an assistant in the Department of Physiology, Faculty of Veterinary Medicine, Atatürk University, Turkey. In 2016, he joined Kafkas University as an assistant professor where he has been engaged in various academic activities. Dr. Gelen has sixty journal articles and twenty poster presentations to his credit. His research interests include physiology, the endocrine system, cancer, diabetes, cardiovascular diseases, and isolated organ bath system studies.

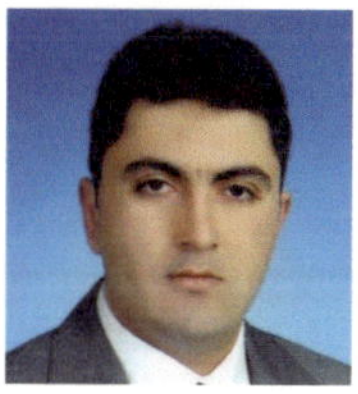

Emin Şengül is a physiology specialist who received his veterinary degree from Atatürk University, Turkey, in 2008. In 2014, he became an assistant professor at the same university. He has published sixty-two journal articles and given twenty poster presentations at scientific congresses. His research interests include physiology, the endocrine system, cancer, diabetes, gastric ulcer, neurotoxicity, testicular toxicity, nephrotoxicity, cardiovascular diseases, and isolated organ bath system studies.

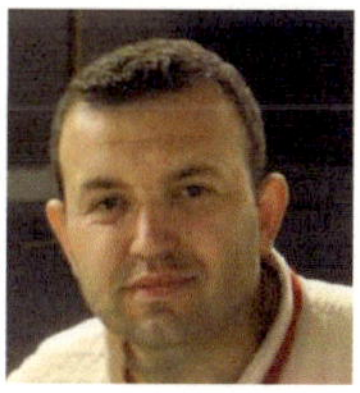

Dr. Abdulsamed Kükürt graduated from Uludağ University, Turkey. In 2019, he obtained a Ph.D. in Biochemistry from the Institute of Health Sciences, Kafkas University, Turkey, where he is currently an assistant professor in the Department of Biochemistry. He has published twenty-eight research articles in academic journals, eleven book chapters, and thirty-seven papers. Dr. Kükürt has participated in ten academic projects and is a reviewer for many academic journals.

Contents

Preface

The hormone melatonin is known as the "hormone of darkness" because it is secreted at night. It has a strong antioxidant capacity as well as immune-boosting, anti-neoplastic, analgesic, and anti-inflammatory effects. As such, it is effective in the treatment of brain and heart diseases and is beneficial for lowering cholesterol and high blood pressure. It also protects against obesity, diabetes, and brain diseases such as Parkinson's, Alzheimer's, dementia, and epilepsy. It supports the immune system and protects it from infections. It also has an anti-aging effect by preventing free radical damage. This book explains the synthesis and regulation of melatonin as well as its antioxidant effects. It examines the hormone's effects on reproductive physiology, Parkinson's, and breast cancer as well as its role in cardiovascular failure and its importance in animal nutrition.

Volkan Gelen
Faculty of Veterinary Medicine,
Department of Physiology,
Kafkas University,
Kars, Turkey

Emin Şengül
Faculty of Veterinary Medicine,
Department of Physiology,
Atatürk University,
Erzurum, Turkey

Abdulsamed Kükürt
Deparment of Biochemistry,
Kafkas University,
Kars, Turkey

Section 1

Melatonin Structure and Synthesis

Chapter 1

Characteristic, Synthesis, and Non-Photic Regulation of Endogenous Melatonin

Mohammed Albreiki

Abstract

Several researchers have confirmed that the melatonin hormone is significant to the body's circadian rhythm, hence, the need to explore the connection between the two aspects. The circadian rhythm is a natural endogenous process that controls essential body functions as it affects hormone release, body temperature, sleep patterns, and eating habits. In that view, the circadian rhythm relies on melatonin to synchronize the night and day cycles. Melatonin plays a significant role in controlling the circadian rhythm by facilitating quality sleep at night and alertness during the day. In effect, understanding the acute non-image-forming visual effects of melatonin will help derive ways to ensure the circadian rhythms operate efficiently for healthy body functions.

Keywords: melatonin, circadian rhythm, non-photic regulation

1. Introduction

Melatonin was discovered in 1958 by an American professor and dermatologist, Aaron B. Lerner, at the Yale University School of Medicine. Lerner and his colleagues were investigating for something that could help in curing skin diseases, which led them to isolate a hormone from bovine pineal gland extracts [1]. The scientists gave the hormone its name due to its property of lightening amphibians' skin pigmentation by inhibiting the melanocyte hormone's skin-darkening aspect. The researchers aimed to use melatonin in curing skin diseases, but in the mid-1970s, they illustrated that the hormone could regulate the circadian rhythm in the pineal glands of living organisms [2, 3]. Specifically, the subsequent years, specifically 1993, also saw extensive research on the hormone, leading to its discovery as an oxidant [3, 4]. Precisely, melatonin discovery began as an investigation of cures to skin diseases, leading to the discovery of its connection with the circadian rhythm. As such, delving into the discovery of melatonin will provide a background to its significance in the circadian rhythm.

1.1 The endogenous hormone melatonin

Endogenous melatonin hormone undergoes various processes in integrating with circadian rhythm to initiate sleep and facilitate several nighttime physiologic functions. Notably, endogenous melatonin is what the body naturally makes instead of exogenous melatonin, which is synthetically produced as a pill, supplement, capsule, or liquid. Melatonin secretion can occur from other body tissues, but the pineal gland, an endocrine gland in the brain, is primarily responsible for secreting the endogenous melatonin [5]. When the optic nerve senses darkness, it sends a signal to the pineal gland, which then responds by releasing melatonin to perform its nighttime functions. Once secreted, endogenous melatonin goes into the bloodstream, and cerebrospinal fluid then begins to send signals to other organs [5]. The circulation then carries the hormone from the brain to the rest of the body, where melatonin receptors detect the rush in circulation and transmit the signal to the body that it is nighttime [6, 7]. In essence, endogenous melatonin production relies on retinal photoreceptors detecting light and darkness and sending signals to the pineal gland [6, 8]. Its circulation to the body then leverages its chemical, making it convenient for distribution [7]. Endogenous melatonin has several chemical properties, and its hydrophilic and lipophilic nature making it easily dissolvable in water and lipids [6]. Besides, the chemical representation of melatonin is N-acetyl-methoxytryptamine, which derives from the processes it undergoes during its synthesis [7]. In short, endogenous melatonin is critical in facilitating essential body functions due to its chemical properties and interaction with other organs. Thus, the endogenous melatonin overview gives an insight into its production and distribution processes, as outlined below.

1.1.1 Melatonin synthesis

Melatonin synthesis occurs through acetylation, methylation, hydroxylation, and decarboxylation. Serotonin, a neurotransmitter from the amino acid tryptophan, is the primary precursor to melatonin [9, 10]. Particularly, L-tryptophan derives from protein catabolism or shikimate pathway from chorismate, then tryptophan hydroxylase hydroxylates it on indole rng to release 5-hydroxytryptophan (5-HTP) [10, 11]. Next, 5-hydroxytryptophan and pyridoxal phosphate decarboxylate the intermediate 5-HTP to form serotonin. Serotonin is initially acetylated and later methylated within the pineal gland to form melatonin [10]. In detail, serotonin *N*-acetyltransferase and acetyl-CoA convert serotonin into *N*-acetylserotonin [12, 13]. *S*-adenosyl methionine and hydroxyindole *O*-methyltransferase form the methylation process to convert *N*-acetylserotonin into melatonin [13, 14]. The process relies on light exposure to optical nerves since the serum concentrations vary with dark and daylight [13]. In essence, serotonin N-acetyltransferase (NAT) is in low concentration during the daytime and rises during the dark, dark-phase [13, 15]. Notably, although the methyltransferase process does not follow the light exposure pattern, it can only take place after the completion of the first-phase. That means melatonin synthesis is dependent on the light-dark cycle for the successful process completion of a biochemical pathway [10, 13, 15]. In the absence of light (nighttime), noradrenaline binds to α and β adrenergic receptors causing an increase in intracellular Ca^{2+}. Intracellular Ca^{2+} increases and potentiate protein kinase C (PKC) and calcium-calmodulin protein kinase (CaM kinase), which in turn increases cAMP and phosphorylation of rate-limiting enzymes in melatonin synthesis (AANAT and HIOMT) (**Figure 1**) [16]. In simple terms, melatonin synthesis is the hydroxylation and decarboxylation of serotoninbased on the changes in the light-dark cycle. That way, assessing melatonin synthesis acts as a basis for understanding melatonin production phases to help treat sleeping disorders.

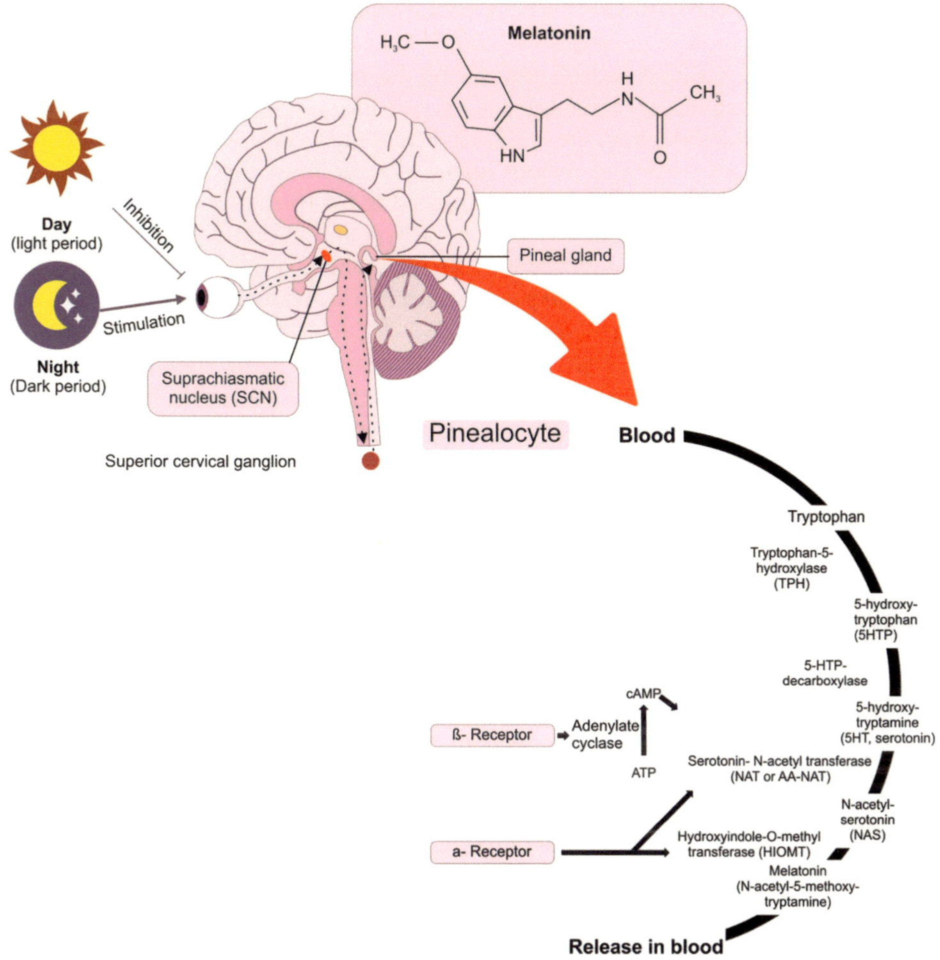

Figure 1.
Melatonin structure and biosynthesis pathway. Schematic representation of melatonin chemical structure, synthesis, and secretion. The hormone melatonin is syntheised from tryptophan with the rate-limiting enzymes, AA-NAT and HIOMT. NEinfluence α and β adrenoreceptors on pinealocytes to enhance the activity of intercellular enzymes needed for meltoning synthesis (Adopted from Watson [16]).

1.1.2 Melatonin catabolism

Melatonin catabolism is the process of metabolism that releases energy to facilitate different body functions. Originally, the body's behavioral and physiological processes aligned to ensure constant energy intake, storage, and usage. Energy is vital because it facilitates human survival, reproduction, growth, and species regeneration. In that light, energy uptake mainly takes place during the day and storage during the night following the effects of the circadian rhythm [16, 17]. Melatonin thus acts as the linkage between energy distribution in the body and the cyclic revolution of the circadian rhythm [16, 17]. The hormone regulates metabolic processes through the concepts of endocrinology and chronobiology, leading to energy balance as the outcome. After its production, melatonin goes to the brain through blood uptake or pineal recess and then undergoes some concurrent pathways to reach its catabolic sites [17, 18]. One of the pathways leads to the mitochondria in different organs where melatonin exists in high concentrations [17, 19]. The hormone thus significantly plays a significant part as a mitochondrial antioxidant due to the high concentrations in the mitochondria, its free radical scavenging characteristic, and its indirect influence on the definition of antioxidant enzymes [17, 18, 20]. Mainly, the precursor to melatonin catabolism is the transmission to various pathways after its synthesis. In effect, exploring the precursor process acts as a basis for understanding melatonin's catabolic phase.

Primarily, melatonin catabolism occurs in the liver and the kidney, where it undergoes chemical processes for energy production. Melatonin mainly undergoes enzymatic and nonenzymatic redox reactions to produce melatonin metabolite. Nonenzymic are propelled by singlet oxygen, free radicals, and additional reactive intermediates, such as peroxynitrite and HOCL [21]. Non-enzymic melatonin metabolism increases with an upsurge to light exposure leading to the release of N1-acetyl-N2-formyl-5-methoxykynuramine (AFMK) and melatonin [20–22]. Conversely, the enzymatic process involves hydroxylation and conjugation into glucuronide and sulfate [21]. The process occurs in the liver where microsomal cytochrome P_{450} monooxygenase (CYP1A2, CYP1A1, or CYP1B1) hydroxylate melatonin to 6-hydroxy-MEL [20, 23]. The end product, 6-hydroxymelatonin, proceeds to conjugate with sulfuric acid via sulfotransferase to form 6-sulfatoxymelatonin (aMT6s) as the primary melatonin metabolite in the kidney [24]. The end product can then be excreted in the urine or catalyzed by UDP-glucuronosyltransferase to form 6-hydroxymelatonin glucuronide [16, 23]. Notably, that makes urine the main component in determining melatonin concentrations and estimating dim light melatonin onset (DLMO) since it accounts for more than 90% of the metabolized melatonin from aMT6s [16]. The bottom line is that the enzymatic and nonenzymatic catalysis products are similar, with minimal evidence of some taxon-site-specific disparities. Therefore, melatonin catabolism acts as the basis for treating sleep disorders by undergoing chemical reactions in the liver and kidney to release melatonin in body fluids, which helps measure concentrations.

1.1.3 Melatonin measurement

Melatonin measurement in humans is critical since it is the basis of treating sleeping disorders by observing different parameters relating to the sleep cycle. Melatonin measurements primarily occur by gauging its concentrations in bioliquids, such as saliva, urine, plasma, and serum [25]. The highest concentrations mainly occur closer to the pineal gland and reduce as it goes further in the body and mixes with other fluids [25]. Besides remaining in the blood and cerebral fluids, the hormone's hydrophilic and lipophilic nature allows it to diffuse easily into other body fluids, including urine, saliva, amniotic fluid, and sperm [5, 6, 25]. From that perspective, melatonin measurement relies on capturing melatonin increase parameters, one of the common ones being the dim-light melatonin onset (DLMO) [26, 27]. Specifically, DLMO facilitates the melatonin measurements in saliva, blood, or urine samples under dim light. Since there is no stipulated approximation protocol for DLMO, sampling largely relies on observation duration, frequency, and customized estimation threshold [28, 29]. Some of the common DLMO estimation models include enzyme-linked immunosorbent assay (ELISA) and radioimmunoassay (RIA) [27, 30]. High-performance liquid chromatography (HPLC) stands as a less recognized threshold, while fast-scan cycle voltammetry (FSCV) is an upcoming viable model [26, 31]. From that view, melatonin measurements rely on different thresholds that measure the DLMO parameter. That way, acknowledging the different thresholds for melatonin measurement provides a broader view of different approaches to treating sleep disorders.

Since RIA and ELISA stand as the most popular melatonin measurement models, it is fundamental to understand their operational processes. RIA primarily measures melatonin levels in blood, urine, and saliva through a quantitative analysis of high specificity and sensitivity [28, 30]. The method derives from radioactivity measurement of the radioisotope and uses labeled melatonin, unlabeled melatonin, and anti-melatonin antibodies. Labeled and unlabeled melatonin contest for antibody-binding points, creating a scenario where the increment of any leads to the decrease of the other. Afterward, the bound antibody-melatonin gets into the solid-phase and separates from unbound melatonin [28, 29]. The radioactivity measure of the bound melatonin thus derives results, where high radioactivity represents low levels and vice versa [27–29]. Conversely, the ELISA model is an immunoenzymatic approach that measures melatonin thresholds in urine, saliva, and blood [26, 28]. The method can operate under different modifications. All rely on impairing the antigen in melatonin's solid-phase and then progressively replacing it with antigen-specific antibodies, forming an antigen-antibody complex. Next, the resultant medium is rinsed and mixed with the correct amount of enzyme-labeled antibody substrate to attain a color reaction [26, 28]. Eventually, the final results derive from the spectrophotometric measurement, which reveals melatonin levels [28, 32]. In that light, the two melatonin measurement models vary in that one relies on radioactivity and the other on color representation. As such, RIA and ELISA melatonin measurement models help cure sleep disorders by gauging the concentration levels of melatonin in the human body.

1.1.4 Distribution of melatonin receptors

Melatonin functions rely on the hormone's receptors, hence, the need to determine their distribution in the human body. Notably, the receptors present different biological effects, such as enhancing the expression of antioxidant enzymes like glutathione peroxidase, catalase, and superoxide dismutase through signal transduction [3, 25]. The primary melatonin receptors are melatonin receptor 1 (Mel 1A or M1) and melatonin receptor 2 (Mel 1B or M2) since they are the most widely distributed in the body [25, 33]. M1 mainly has a picomolar binding affinity, and M2 is a nanomolar binding activity with the two receptors falling in G-protein coupled receptors (GPCES) [25]. Other receptors include nuclear orphan receptors in retinoid Z receptors (RZR) or retinoid orphan receptors (RORα) family, as well as quinone reductase II enzyme (MT3 receptor) [34–36]. Melatonin receptors derive from different tissues, with the highest density expressed from the suprachiasmatic nucleus, retina, and anterior pituitary [25, 34]. From there, they are vastly distributed in the body to enable their biological functions and expression, as illustrated in the table and chart below [37, 38]. Precisely, melatonin receptors consist of M1, M2, MT3, and orphan receptors, which have varying distribution in the body. Thus, assessing the distribution of melatonin receptors will help determine the treatments for sleep disorders (**Figure 2** and **Table 1**).

1.2 Circadian rhythm

The circadian rhythm is one of the body's biological rhythms and comprises a series of body operations under the influence of the biological clock or internal clock. Biological rhythms range from short ones that take 24 hours to long ones that

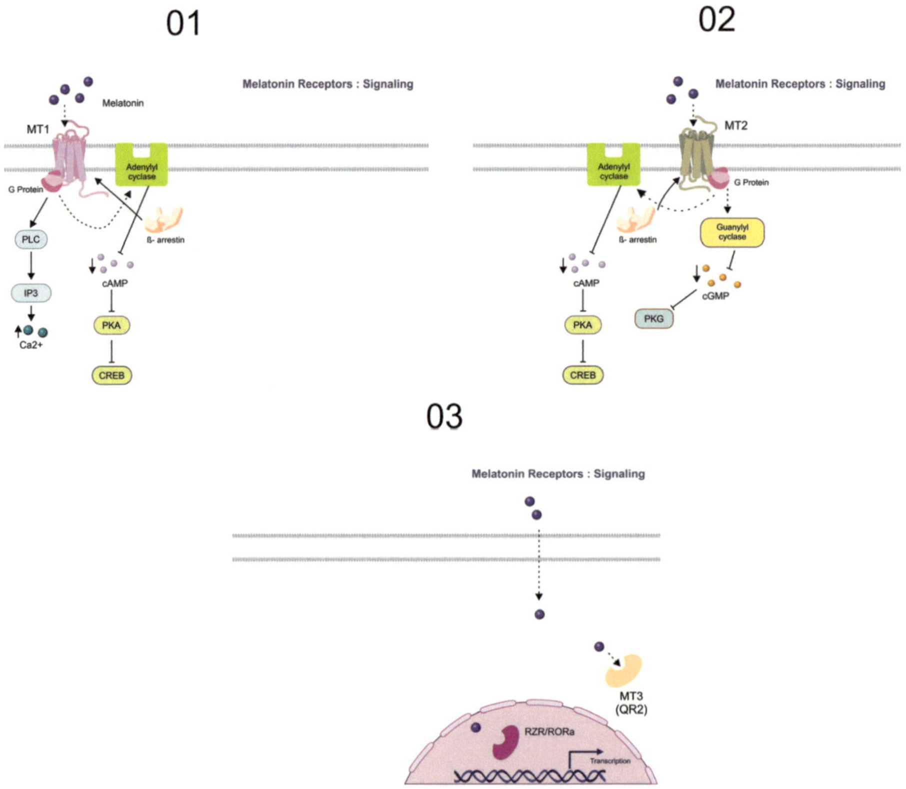

Figure 2.
Major types of melatonin receptors. cAMP and inositol triphosphate (IP3) are the majorintracellular messengers' targets of MT1 and MT2. MT3 targets cytosolic quinone reductase-2 and PORa/RZR1 are the major nuclear receptors formelatonin (Adopted from Tarocco et al. [38]).

Mel receptors	Distributions
MT_1	SCN, cerebellum, hippocampus, retina, ovary, testis, aorta, coronary blood vessels, liver, kidney, adrenal gland, immune system, skin, and gallbladder.
MT_2	SCN, cerebellum, hippocampus, retina, lung, heart, duodenum, granulosa, and adipocytes.
MT_3	Liver, kidney, brain, heart, lung, intestine, muscle, brown adipose tissue, and eye.
MT_4	Brain, pineal and neurons, and spinal cord.

Table list the subtypes of melatonin receptors. MT1 and MT2 are widely distributed in mammalian tissues (Adapted from [16, 25, 38]).

Table 1.
Distribution of melatonin receptors.

go up to a year [39]. The dominant biological rhythms include the circadian, diurnal, infradian, circalunar, and circannual, with the circadian being a 24-hour cycle. Circadian rhythms are critical because they regulate several body cycles, including sleep, alertness, hormone production, and body temperature, and their interruption may present mild to severe disorders [39, 40]. They derive from natural body factors, with the main ones being cryptochrome and period genes, which code for protein build-up in the cell's nucleus with the light-dark cycle [39, 41–43]. Nevertheless, various molecular chemicals can sustain or disrupt the circadian rhythm based on light exposure, environmental cues, prescription drugs, exercise, and eating habits [44–46]. The factors mainly affect circadian rhythms and cause disorders by breaking the connection with the internal clock. The suprachiasmatic nucleus (SCN) in the brain's hypothalamus is the internal clock responsible for controlling the circadian rhythm [44, 47, 48]. SCN's main role is to regulate the pituitary gland and the autonomic nervous system by transmitting signals to manage body activity [44]. Precisely, the process takes place with the intervention of MT1 and MT2 receptors as they help induce the beneficial outcomes of melatonin in correcting sleep disorders. In effect, delving into the circadian rhythm background will guide into understanding its connection with endogenous melatonin.

1.2.1 Circadian rhythm of endogenous melatonin

The everyday sleep-wake cycle relies on the actions of the internal clock and the homeostatic sleep process driven by circadian rhythm and endogenous melatonin. The circadian rhythm is the leading facilitator of endogenous melatonin production following the daily oscillation of internal clock genes throughout the day [49, 50]. Melatonin exhibits a clear circadian rhythm property, as evident from the hormone's synthesis and secretion mechanism. Despite the presence of non-photic stimuli, such as food, temperature, rest-activity schedule in entertaining circadian rhythm, and the light-dark cycle, is considered as the strongest zeitgeber. From that perspective, light exposure to the retina is immediately transmitted to the suprachiasmatic nuclei, which inhibits melatonin production during the day, by transmitting inhibitory signals to the pineal gland [49]. Melatonin synthesis and secretion have a rhythmic pattern, as the amplitude of secretion (acrophase) is the highest between 02:00 and 04:00h, and the concentration of serum melatonin at night reaches 8-120 pg/ml [50, 51]. The activity of rate-limiting enzymes, AANAT, and HIOMT, found at the highest concentration during the dark hours [52–55]. The bottom line, light is the central controller of the circadian clock by triggering the activity of the suprachiasmatic clock, which sends signals to the pineal gland for melatonin production. That way, the circadian rhythm is a component of endogenous melatonin, and the two are involved in various body functions based on the reactions of the internal clock.

1.2.2 Melatonin as a marker of circadian phase

Melatonin is the primary marker of the circadian rhythm as it advances the circadian rhythms with changes in the light-dark cycle. It is a chronobiotic molecule or known as the hormone of darkness as it signals the length of night and time of day/year in all tissues. Its potential to cause phase-advance or phasedelay has been proven when administered at a different time of the day [16, 56]. The evening increment in melatonin influences changes in objective markers of drowsiness, including slow eye movement, slow eyeblink rate, and sleep epochs [57]. Melatonin thus acts as a phase marker based on its profile composition, which includes melatonin onset, acrophase or peak time, melatonin mid-range, and mid-range cross [57]. Notably, DLMO is the core element that gives melatonin its property as a marker of the circadian rhythm as it controls the processes of melatonin onset and offset [58]. Additionally, it influences melatonin concentrations across different types of daylight and nighttime, initiating sleep or other biological processes [58]. In a nutshell, melatonin as the main marker coordinates with other circadian phase markers to initiate the sleep cycle and other body functions. Thus, melatonin as a circadian phase marker helps treat sleep disorders by integrating different components of the circadian rhythm.

1.3 Non-Photic factors affecting Endogenous melatonin

Non-photic factors that range from lifestyle preferences, including dietary intake, nicotine, caffeine, and alcohol, or even physiological changes, including menstrual cycle, drugs, and changes in posture, can potentially regulate melatonin rhythms and levels. Hence, it is essential to focus on other factors during the experimental protocol and design to ensure robust and consistent outcomes, including minimizing the possibility of certain confounding factors. Such factors are illustrated below:

1.3.1 Dietary intake

A number of human studies have associated changes in energy restriction and dietary intake with melatonin concentration or synthesis. Some studies reported a 20% melatonin reduction after an energy intake of more than 300 Kcal every day from 2–7 days, with insignificant change in the AMT6s in the human urine [59, 60]. The levels maintained to normal after supplementation of glucose in the short term show that pinealocytes need glucose delivery to function appropriately [60]. Essentially, melatonin has been significantly found in substantive amounts in vegetables, including barley, walnuts, tomatoes, rice, and olives [61]. For example, taking vegetables in the morning has been linked to the higher excretion of urinary aMT6s [62, 63]. There were similar statistics in Japanese women, where a similar increased mean for the urinary aMT6s in a high intake of vegetables than the ones with the lowest consumption, essentially by 16% [59, 64].

The increasing level of melatonin is more likely to result from the stimulatory effects of the consumed products instead of the absorbed dietary food enriched with melatonin [65, 66]. Melatonin is usually found in milk products, especially those produced during the night [62, 67]. Therefore, it is imperative to conclude that nighttime lactation has been associated with various physiological importance attached to it as part of the infant's diet [61]. Nevertheless, St. Hilaire et al. [68] adds that the possibility of maternal melatonin passing via the milk to the infant leads to enhanced nocturnal sleep [59]. Moreover, sleep parameters improvement and greater urinary metabolites of serotonin were observed in the intake of TRP-enriched commercial milk by the infants. The Figure below demonstrates different changes in levels of maternal salivary melatonin at night time in normal pregnancy.

According to Ahammed et al. [63], the relationship between melatonin levels and the availability of nutrients in urine and plasma was observed in animal research [66, 67]. Further, in rodents, the registered decrease in plasma melatonin was linked with zinc, folate, and magnesium deficiency in mice [61]. B6 vitamin and folate usually serve as the required coenzyme information of serotonin from TRP, while magnesium and zinc, on the other hand, increase AANAT affinity in bond formation with serotonin as well as melatonin formation [61]. Many human studies showed a lack of correlation between the minerals, including zinc, magnesium, and folate, or vitamins, with variations in melatonin in urine or plasma [65].

1.3.2 Posture

Ahammed et al. [63] affirm that different changes have linked postures changes in humans with cardiac autonomic drive. Further studies show variations in heart rate between the sitting and supine, standing and supine, standing, supine and head-down tilt, and head-up postures [60, 65]. The variations in the autonomic balance were observed with the changes in posture from supine vertical sitting or standing posture [60]. Changing posture usually affects the blood volume since there is redistribution of blood during changes in posture, particularly from supine to standing [69]. Studies have suggested a significant variation in the antigravity muscle activities once there are changes in posture, and the muscles are critical in the vascular and vasomotor activity [60, 62].

Nonetheless, these explanations and observations raise a question about the possibility of any variation in the melatonin levels, including saliva, plasma, and urine, via various postures [65]. Salivary and plasma melatonin decreased while moving from the supine to the standing posture and was raised during the reversal of the positions [69, 70]. Additionally, different studies added that raised levels of plasma melatonin during a sitting posture but did not observe any difference in the position change from sitting to the standing posture [64]. On the contrary, recent studies reported raised levels of salivary melatonin during standing posture than in sitting position after collecting samples at midnight but did not observe any difference about 35 minutes ago [70].

1.3.3 Physical activity

St. Hilaire et al. [68] argue that it is controversial how physical exercises can influence endogenous melatonin, although most studies suggest that increased exercise has the potential to influence and regulate endogenous melatonin in two distinct ways: influencing the melatonin rhythm and regulating melatonin levels in physiological fluids [68, 70].

Studies by Kirsz et al. have provided substantive evidence that exercising during night hours has great potential to increase delays in the onset of melatonin [71]. This study was also reported with higher and moderate-intensity/regularly in dim light or dark conditions, including old and younger participants [70]. Further studies report that there is usually rare exercise-induced advance. Nevertheless, further studies observed a phase advance during morning hours than during evening and nighttime exercises [64, 69].

Additionally, exercises have been found to alter/change melatonin levels accurately because of their phase-shifting effects. Following an exercise bout, circulating melatonin was reported to have increased transiently [60]. Nonetheless, this short increase was attributed to vigorous regular training or the progression of regular exercises, including treadmill research [64].

Research has shown increased sympathetic nervous system and secretion of catecholamine, induced by exercises, which can potentially control secretion. Further, exercises have been found to stimulate MRN (midbrain raphe nuclei) that transmits serotoninergic signals to the IGL [72]. The latter can potentially link SCN through NPY release [70]. Also, MRN depends on arousal since the serotonin levels in SCN follow the routine trend of locomotor activity in both nocturnal and diurnal rodents. Because serotonin can indirectly and directly affect SCN, it informs that the ability to enhance mood can be due to its potential in resetting SCN.

1.3.4 Menstrual cycle

According to Minella et al., variations in melatonin levels have been identified across the phases of menstruation. Therefore, increased plasma melatonin was seen in women in LP (luteal-phase) than FP (follicular-phase) [73]. There was also an increase in the melatonin levels in the participants taking a three-phase contraceptive pill. Most of these findings were supported by increased urinary aMT6s during LP [72]. Nonetheless, a one-day area under the plasma melatonin curve was greatly reduced in LP without changes in timing measures as illustrated below [70]. This, therefore, shows a possibility of interaction between melatonin and progesterone, including melatonin serving as a modulator of menstrual phases [66].

Moreover, evidence from studies suggests that the interaction of melatonin and sex hormones results from localizing melatonin receptors with progesterone and estrogen in the periphery and brain, including the increased melatonin receptors in the reproductive tissues [70, 73]. The study also reported a marked increase in melatonin secretion in women using oral contraceptives, particularly synthetic progesterone, as well as melatonin treatment could be essential in enhancing human chronic gonadotropin-stimulated progesterone secretion in human granulosa cells [73]. In contrast, in a low estrogen environment and premenopausal women, oophorectomy contributes to substantially increased melatonin secretion [74].

Further, Gentry et al. [75] add that treating estrogen was found to significantly reduce melatonin synthesis in rat pinealocytes, with reduced melatonin receptors (MTI) being further seen in ovaries in rats [72, 75]. Patients with PMDD (premenstrual dysphoric disorder) have been found to have reduced serotonin levels with changes in timing and the amount of secreted nocturnal melatonin [74]. This finding, however, raises the question of how reduced serotonin, which is the precursor of melatonin synthesis, can change the production of melatonin in the pineal gland Pevet et al. [66].

1.3.5 Alcohol

Studies conducted by Hardeland [76] shows that beer and wine with identical amounts of melatonin can potentially influence melatonin level in body fluids. Nonetheless, the influence of chronic or acute consumption of alcohol on levels of melatonin is inconsistent [74, 76]. Social drinking, such as 10–100g of ethanol daily, was found to decrease levels of melatonin in the blood [74]. In another study that involved heavy consumption of beer, 24–48g of ethanol in females and males resulted in a significant rise in serum melatonin following the high content of melatonin in beer [66, 70]. Contrary, repeated or single routine doses of between 15 and 120g ethanol was established to reduce aMT6s over a one-day period with more doses of alcohol [21, 77]. Similar results involved a categorical analysis showed no effect of a single drink, with two drinks leading to a 9% decline, 15% with 3, and 17% reduction with four or more drinks [70]. The above studies considered such factors as medication use, age, and hours of darkness.

1.3.6 Caffeine

Despite a standard cup of coffee was projected to have 40 μg of melatonin, the role of caffeine in the circulation of melatonin concentration remains unclear [69]. Other clinical studies show that a dose of 200 mg of caffeine capsules results in a decrease in the secretion of nocturnal secretion, with another study showing an increase of around 32% in plasma melatonin [77, 78]. A decrease of 7% in the nocturnal melatonin was identified in the healthy young participants after the administration of 400 mg caffeine was repeated at an interval of one week. In similar research, when the participants took coffee, an observation was made that a decline of over 49% night-time aMT6s excretion in a coffee with caffeine than in the coffee without caffeine [69]. Essentially, caffeine was found to serve as an adenosine antagonist inhibiting intracellular cAMP activity, hence, the production of AANAT.

1.3.7 Drugs

Sharafi et al. (2019) argue that drugs, including prescribed, recreational, and conventional ones, have been found to contain different effects on melatonin secretion and synthesis. Atenolol has been linked to significant light-induced phase delays in the onset of melatonin in humans [78]. Psychotropic and antidepressant drugs have been associated with changes in pineal functions and melatonin levels, as shown in **Figure 1** [62, 69]. Various types of selective serotonin inhibitors, SSRI, including fluvoxamine, result in a notable rise in plasma melatonin concentrations. While others, including citalopram, showed no effect. Minella et al. (2021) add that tricyclic antidepressants enhance the onset of melatonin and intensify the nocturnal plasma melatonin in people since it acts as noradrenaline re-uptake inhibitors [73].

1.3.8 Nicotine

Cigarettes usually contain polycyclic aromatic hydrocarbons that usually contain CYP1A2 activity, which is required for the metabolism of melatonin in the liver [62, 73]. Therefore, the level of melatonin in habitual smokers is usually low. Administration of chronic nicotine contributes to increased CYP1A2 levels as well enzymatic activity. Such observations were seen in greater amounts in smokers [72, 74]. After experiments were done on smokers prior to and after smoking abstinence have shown changes in endogenous levels of melatonin; however, after administration of oral melatonin (usually 25 mg) during the night, levels of melatonin during the period without smoking were substantially higher than during smoking period [72, 78].

2. Conclusion

Melatonin hormone is a critical component in treating sleep and other body disorders arising from the disruption of the circadian rhythm. Melatonin comes as an endogenous or exogenous hormone, where endogenous derives naturally from the body and exogenous is manufactured in the laboratory. With respect to endogenous melatonin, it derives from the pineal glands in the brain and undergoes various processes before attaining its ultimate outcomes. Particularly, melatonin undergoes biosynthesis and catabolism, and the metabolites are distributed throughout the body to different types of receptors. Melatonin concentration measurement thus becomes possible by testing the end products from different sites using gauging models, such as RIA and ELISA. The essence of understanding melatonin demographics is mainly to connect its connection with the circadian rhythm in facilitating body cycles. Precisely, the melatonin hormone undergoes its processes in resonance with the circadian rhythm for it to complete its physiological pathways. Therefore, exploring the connection between melatonin production and circadian rhythms helps understand the body's physiological processes in contracting or treating sleep disorders. Conclusively, every non-photic factor has been found to have a significant effect on endogenous melatonin. Several studies have exhausted the effects including increase or decrease of melatonin levels upon experiments on the different non-photic factors.

Author details

Mohammed Albreiki
Center for Biotechnology, Khalifa University of Science and Technology, Abu Dhabi, United Arab Emirates

*Address all correspondence to: mohammed.albreiki@wsu.ede

References

[1] Lerner AB et al. Isolation of melatonin, the pineal gland factor that lightens melanocyteS1. Journal of the American Chemical Society. 1958;**80**(10):2587-2587

[2] Anton-Tay F, Diaz J, Fernandez-Guardiola A. On the effect of melatonin upon human brain. Its possible therapeutic implications. Life Sciences. 1971;**10**(15):841-850

[3] Cipolla-Neto J, Amaral FGD. Melatonin as a hormone: New physiological and clinical insights. Endocrine Reviews. 2018;**39**(6):990-1028

[4] Hardeland R et al. The significance of the metabolism of the neurohormone melatonin: Antioxidative protection and formation of bioactive substances. Neuroscience & Biobehavioral Reviews. 1993;**17**(3):347-357

[5] Yu H-S, Tsin AT, Reiter RJ. Melatonin: History, biosynthesis, and assay methodology. In: Melatonin. USA: CRC Press; 2020. pp. 1-16

[6] Caniato R et al. Melatonin in plants. In: Developments in Tryptophan and Serotonin Metabolism. Poland: Springer; 2003. pp. 593-597

[7] Hacışevki A, Baba B. An overview of melatonin as an antioxidant molecule: A biochemical approach. Melatonin molecular biology. Clinical and Pharmaceutical Approaches. 2018;**5**:59-85

[8] Macchi MM, Bruce JN. Human pineal physiology and functional significance of melatonin. Frontiers in Neuroendocrinology. 2004;**25**(3-4):177-195

[9] Hardeland R. Melatonin in plants and other phototrophs: Advances and gaps concerning the diversity of functions. Journal of Experimental Botany. 2015;**66**(3):627-646

[10] Zhao D et al. Melatonin synthesis and function: Evolutionary history in animals and plants. Frontiers in Endocrinology. 2019;**10**:249

[11] Tan DX et al. On the significance of an alternate pathway of melatonin synthesis via 5-methoxytryptamine: Comparisons across species. Journal of Pineal Research. 2016;**61**(1):27-40

[12] Ye T et al. Metabolic analysis of the melatonin biosynthesis pathway using chemical labeling coupled with liquid chromatography-mass spectrometry. Journal of Pineal Research. 2019;**66**(1):e12531

[13] Xie X et al. Melatonin biosynthesis pathways in nature and its production in engineered microorganisms. Synthetic and Systems Biotechnology. 2022;7(1):544-553

[14] Wang S-Y, Shi X-C, Laborda P. Indole-based melatonin analogues: Synthetic approaches and biological activity. European Journal of Medicinal Chemistry. 2020;**185**:111847

[15] Ackermann K, Stehle JH. Melatonin synthesis in the human pineal gland: Advantages, implications, and difficulties. Chronobiology International. 2006;**23**(1-2):369-379

[16] Watson RR. Melatonin in the Promotion of Health. USA: CRC Press; 2011

[17] Slominski AT et al. Melatonin: A cutaneous perspective on its

production, metabolism, and functions. Journal of Investigative Dermatology. 2018;**138**(3):490-499

[18] Acuña-Castroviejo D et al. Extrapineal melatonin: Sources, regulation, and potential functions. Cellular and Molecular Life Sciences. 2014;**71**(16):2997-3025

[19] Huo X et al. Human transporters, PEPT 1/2, facilitate melatonin transportation into mitochondria of cancer cells: An implication of the therapeutic potential. Journal of Pineal Research. 2017;**62**(4):e12390

[20] Hardeland R. Taxon-and site-specific melatonin catabolism. Molecules. 2017;**22**(11):2015

[21] Hardeland R. Melatonin, its metabolites and their interference with reactive nitrogen compounds. Molecules. 2021;**26**(13):4105

[22] Yasui-Furukori N et al. Association between cytochrome P450 (CYP) 2C19 polymorphisms and harm avoidance in Japanese. American Journal of Medical Genetics Part B: Neuropsychiatric Genetics. 2007;**144**(6):724-727

[23] Ma X et al. Metabolism of melatonin by human cytochromes p450. Drug Metabolism and Disposition. 2005;**33**(4):489-494

[24] Ma X et al. A metabolomic perspective of melatonin metabolism in the mouse. Endocrinology. 2008;**149**(4):1869-1879

[25] Oishi A, Gbahou F, Jockers R. Melatonin receptors, brain functions, and therapies. Handbook of Clinical Neurology. 2021;**179**:345-356

[26] Kennaway DJ. A critical review of melatonin assays: Past and present. Journal of Pineal Research. 2019;**67**(1):e12572

[27] Kennaway DJ. Measuring melatonin by immunoassay. Journal of Pineal Research. 2020;**69**(1):e12657

[28] Rzepka-Migut B, Paprocka J. Melatonin-measurement methods and the factors modifying the results. A systematic review of the literature. International Journal of Environmental Research and Public Health. 2020;**17**(6):1916

[29] De Almeida EA et al. Measurement of melatonin in body fluids: Standards, protocols and procedures. Child's Nervous System. 2011;**27**(6):879-891

[30] Middleton B. Measurement of melatonin and 6-sulphatoxymelatonin. In: Hormone Assays in Biological Fluids. USA: Springer; 2013. pp. 171-199

[31] Martinez GR et al. Measurement of melatonin and its metabolites. Endocrine. 2005;**27**(2):111-118

[32] Kennaway DJ. Measuring morning melatonin levels with plasma melatonin ELISA kits is a poor choice on two levels. Journal of Pineal Research. 2022;**72**(1):e12773

[33] Liu J et al. MT1 and MT2 melatonin receptors: A therapeutic perspective. Annual Review of Pharmacology and Toxicology. 2016;**56**:361

[34] Jockers R et al. Update on melatonin receptors: IUPHAR Review 20. British Journal of Pharmacology. 2016;**173**(18):2702-2725

[35] Ekmekcioglu C. Melatonin receptors in humans: Biological role and clinical relevance. Biomedicine & Pharmacotherapy. 2006;**60**(3):97-108

[36] Slominski RM et al. Melatonin membrane receptors in peripheral

tissues: Distribution and functions. Molecular and Cellular Endocrinology. 2012;**351**(2):152-166

[37] Wiechmann AF, Sherry DM. Neurotransmitters and Receptors: Melatonin Receptors. Netherlands. 2017

[38] Tarocco A et al. Melatonin as a master regulator of cell death and inflammation: Molecular mechanisms and clinical implications for newborn care. Cell Death & Disease. 2019;**10**(4):1-12

[39] Lu Q, Kim JY. Mammalian circadian networks mediated by the suprachiasmatic nucleus. The FEBS Journal. 2021

[40] Honma S. The mammalian circadian system: A hierarchical multi-oscillator structure for generating circadian rhythm. The Journal of Physiological Sciences. 2018;**68**(3):207-219

[41] Tei H et al. Circadian oscillation of a mammalian homologue of the Drosophila period gene. Nature. 1997;**389**(6650):512-516

[42] Ikeda M, Nomura M. cDNA cloning and tissue-specific expression of a novel basic helix–loop–helix/PAS protein (BMAL1) and identification of alternatively spliced variants with alternative translation initiation site usage. Biochemical and Biophysical Research Communications. 1997;**233**(1):258-264

[43] Kume K et al. mCRY1 and mCRY2 are essential components of the negative limb of the circadian clock feedback loop. Cell. 1999;**98**(2):193-205

[44] Walker WH et al. Circadian rhythm disruption and mental health. Translational Psychiatry. 2020;**10**(1):1-13

[45] Edition F. Diagnostic and statistical manual of mental disorders. American Psychiatric Association. 2013;**21**(21):591-643

[46] Bedrosian T, Nelson R. Timing of light exposure affects mood and brain circuits. Translational Psychiatry. 2017;7(1):e1017-e1017

[47] Partch CL, Green CB, Takahashi JS. Molecular architecture of the mammalian circadian clock. Trends in Cell Biology. 2014;**24**(2):90-99

[48] Takahashi JS. Molecular components of the circadian clock in mammals. Diabetes, Obesity and Metabolism. 2015;**17**:6-11

[49] Vasey C, McBride J, Penta K. Circadian rhythm dysregulation and restoration: The role of melatonin. Nutrients. 2021;**13**(10):3480

[50] Hardeland R et al. Melatonin, the circadian multioscillator system and health: The need for detailed analyses of peripheral melatonin signaling. Journal of Pineal Research. 2012;**52**(2):139-166

[51] Arendt J. Melatonin and the Mammalian Pineal Gland. UK: Springer Science & Business Media; 1994

[52] Besseau L et al. Melatonin pathway: Breaking the 'high-at-night'rule in trout retina. Experimental Eye Research. 2006;**82**(4):620-627

[53] Srinivasan V. Melatonin, oxidative stress and ageing. Current Science. 1999;**76**:46-54

[54] Klein DC. Photoneural regulation of the mammalian pineal gland. Photoperiodism, melatonin and the pineal. 1985;**117**:38-56

[55] Kim T-D et al. Rhythmic control of AANAT translation by hnRNP Q in

circadian melatonin production. Genes & Development. 2007;**21**(7):797-810

[56] Turek FW. Circadian rhythms: From the bench to the bedside and falling asleep. Sleep. 2004;**27**(8):1600-1602

[57] Zerbini G, Winnebeck EC, Merrow M. Weekly, seasonal, and chronotype-dependent variation of dim-light melatonin onset. Journal of Pineal Research. 2021;**70**(3):e12723

[58] Lewy AJ, Sack RL, Singer CM. Immediate and delayed effects of bright light on human melatonin production: Shifting "Dawn" and "Dusk" Shifts the Dim Light Melatonin Onset (DLMO) a. Annals of the New York Academy of Sciences. 1985;**453**(1):253-259

[59] Emens JS et al. Behaviorally and environmentally induced non–24-hour sleep-wake rhythm disorder in sighted patients. Journal of Clinical Sleep Medicine. 2022;**18**(2):453-459

[60] Grant LK et al. Endogenous circadian regulation and phase resetting of clinical metabolic biomarkers. Journal of Pineal Research. 2021;**71**(2):e12752

[61] Liampas I et al. Endogenous melatonin levels and therapeutic use of exogenous melatonin in migraine: Systematic review and meta-analysis. Headache: The Journal of Head and Face Pain. 2020;**60**(7):1273-1299

[62] Soni SK, Kumar D, Singaravel M. Melatonin-induced phase and dose responses in a diurnal mammal. Funambulus pennantii. Chronobiology International. 2020;**37**(5):641-651

[63] Ahammed GJ et al. Endogenous melatonin deficiency aggravates high temperature-induced oxidative stress in Solanum lycopersicum L. Environmental and Experimental Botany. 2019;**161**:303-311

[64] Coirolo N, et al. Non-Photic Modulations of the Circadian Phase of Dancers Trained in Shifts. Netherlands. 2022

[65] Datta K. Biological rhythm and neuropsychiatric disorders. In: Sleep and Neuropsychiatric Disorders. Germany: Springer; 2022. pp. 53-63

[66] Pevet P, Challet E, Felder-Schmittbuhl M-P. Melatonin and the circadian system: Keys for health with a focus on sleep. Handbook of Clinical Neurology. 2021;**179**:331-343

[67] Hu N et al. Daily cycle of melatonin in different tissues of dybowski's frog (Rana dybowskii). Biological Rhythm Research. 2021;**53**:1-9

[68] Hilaire S et al. Prediction of individual differences in circadian adaptation to night work among older adults: Application of a mathematical model using individual sleep-wake and light exposure data. Chronobiology International. 2020;**37**(9-10):1404

[69] Mendoza-Vargas L et al. Involvement of melatonin in the regulation of the Circadian System in Crayfish. International Journal of Molecular Sciences. 2018;**19**(7):2147

[70] Yasmin F et al. Gut melatonin: A potent candidate in the diversified journey of melatonin research. General and Comparative Endocrinology. 2021;**303**:113693

[71] Kirsz K et al. Involvement of orexin A in nocturnal melatonin secretion into the cerebrospinal fluid and the blood plasma in seasonal sheep. General and Comparative Endocrinology. 2020;**286**:113304

[72] Qian J et al. Unanticipated daytime melatonin secretion on a simulated night shift schedule generates a distinctive 24-h melatonin rhythm with antiphasic daytime and nighttime peaks. Journal of Pineal Research. 2022;**72**(3):e12791

[73] Minella C et al. Protective role of melatonin in breast cancer: What we can learn from women with blindness. Cancer Causes & Control. 2021;**33**:1-13

[74] Woodford EC et al. Endogenous melatonin and sleep in individuals with Rare Genetic Neurodevelopmental Disorders (RGND): A systematic review. Sleep Medicine Reviews. 2021;**57**:101433

[75] Gentry NW et al. Human circadian variations. Journal of Clinical Investigation. 2021;**131**(16):e148282

[76] Hardeland R. Divergent importance of chronobiological considerations in high-and low-dose melatonin therapies. Diseases. 2021;**9**(1):18

[77] Choi H, Rao MC, Chang EB. Gut microbiota as a transducer of dietary cues to regulate host circadian rhythms and metabolism. Nature Reviews Gastroenterology & Hepatology. 2021;**18**(10):679-689

[78] Sharafi Y et al. Melatonin treatment promotes endogenous melatonin accumulation and triggers GABA shunt pathway activity in tomato fruits during cold storage. Scientia Horticulturae. 2019;**254**:222-227

Section 2

Effect of Melatonin on Reproduction

Chapter 2

An Overview of Effects on Reproductive Physiology of Melatonin

Volkan Gelen, Emin Şengül and Abdulsamed Kükürt

Abstract

Melatonin is a neurotransmitter released from the pineal gland. The presence of receptor sites in the hypothalamus, pituitary gland, ovaries, and testicles and secretion of pituitary hormones (FSH and LH) are some of the effects of this hormone on reproduction. In addition to its systemic effect, it also showed an effect on ovarian physiology with the detection of high levels in the follicular fluid and the presence of melatonin receptors in the ovarian cells. In addition, it has been determined that melatonin affects follicular growth, oocyte maturation, ovulation, and luteal function. It has been stated that the effects of melatonin on the male reproductive system are indirectly effective through the gonads and indirectly by affecting the hormones. Again, some studies have expressed that melatonin has strong antioxidant properties and affects reproductive physiology due to this effect. This section discusses the effect of melatonin on male and female reproductive physiology.

Keywords: melatonin, reproduction, physiology, FSH, LH, ovarium, testes, oxidative stress

1. Introduction

Melatonin is a hormone secreted by the pineal gland and is known to be involved in the regulation of many body functions and the regulation of circadian and seasonal rhythms [1]. This hormone is rhythmically released from the epiphysis at night [2]. Since its release is regulated according to the nighttime, its secretion occurs with the internal reflection of the external photoperiod [3]. Melatonin is also called the "hormone of darkness". It has been determined that melatonin is synthesized in the lacrimal gland, retina, erythrocytes, platelets, and some cells in the gastrointestinal tract other than the pineal gland, but this synthesis has little effect on the plasma melatonin level [4–7]. The main synthesis site of melatonin is pinealocytes, and it is synthesized from tryptophan in these cells. Tryptophan is first converted to 5-hydroxytryptophan by the enzyme tryptophan hydroxylase. Then 5-hydroxytryptophan is converted to serotonin by amino acid decarboxylase. Serotonin is converted to N-acetyl serotonin by the enzyme N-acetyl transferase. N-acetyl serotonin is converted to melatonin by the enzyme methyltransferase. Thus, the synthesized melatonin is released into the blood circulation [8, 9]. Around 19.00–20.00, melatonin secretion begins to increase, reaches its highest point between 02.00 and 04.00 at night, and decreases with the increase of daylight in the morning. It starts to decrease between 07.00 and 09.00 in the morning [10–12]. Melatonin takes part in many biological and physiological regulations in the body. It is effective on biorhythm (circadian rhythm) and also has direct and indirect effects on the reproductive system, regenerating our cells, regulating the immune system, anticarcinogen, antioxidant, antiaging, and reproductive system [13]. This chapter, it is aimed to explain the physiological effects of melatonin, which has important bodily effects in the body, on the female and male reproductive systems.

2. Melatonin synthesis

Melatonin is synthesized from tryptophan in pinealocytes in the pineal gland. Synthesis stages are, respectively: Tryptophan is converted to 5-hydroxytryptophan by the enzyme tryptophan hydroxylase. Then 5-hydroxytryptophan is converted to serotonin by the amino acid decarboxylase enzyme. Serotonin is converted to N-acetyl serotonin by the enzyme N-acetyl transferase. N-acetyl serotonin is converted to melatonin by the enzyme methyltransferase. Thus, the synthesized melatonin is released into the blood circulation [8, 9]. The regulation of melatonin synthesis is controlled by the retinohypothalamic pathway and a system that surrounds the suprachiasmatic nuclei and contains multiple synapses within this pathway. Stimuli from the retina reach the hypothalamus and then this information reaches the pineal gland via peripheral postganglionic sympathetic fibers and melatonin is synthesized [9]. It activates protein kinase C (PKC) via β- and α1-adrenergic receptors on pinealocytes with increased norepinephrine stimulation at night. PKC activation increases the Ca^{2+} movement in the cell, resulting in an increase in the concentration of intracellular cyclic adenosine monophosphate (cAMP). This increase activates protein kinase A (PKA) (**Figures 1** and **2**). Activated PKA increases AANAT activity [14]. Once synthesized, it is directly secreted into the cerebrospinal fluid and blood of the third ventricle and reaches all body tissues in a very short time. After melatonin is released, it is transported by diffusion and some carrier molecules [15]. Melatonin can regulate a variety of physiological functions, from the well-known modulation of sleep/wake cycles and circadian rhythms to the maintenance and regulation of neural development and immune system and endocrine functions [16]. These effects of the melatonin are mediated by G protein-linked melatonin receptors MT1 and MT2. In addition, activation of a putative cytoplasmic melatonin receptor MT3 is also effective [17]. When melatonin binds to these receptors, due to the connection between the

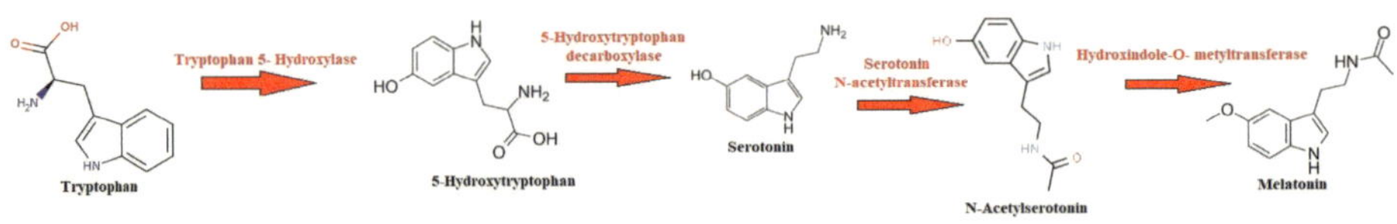

Figure 1.
Biosynthetic pathway of the melatonin.

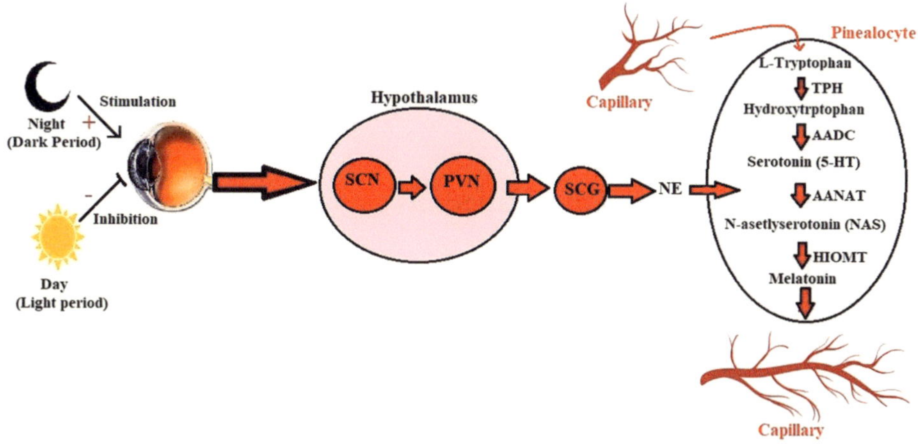

Figure 2.
Synthesis of melatonin from tryptophan under the influence of light in the pineal gland [9]. SCG: Superior cervical ganglion; SCN: Suprachiasmatic nucleus; NA: Noradrenaline; PVN: Paraventricular nucleus; AADC: Aromatic-L-amino-acid decarboxylase AANAT: Arylalkylamine N-acetyltransferase, TPH: Hydroxytryptophan 5-hydroxylase. HIOMT: Hydroxy indole-O-methyltransferase NAS: N-asetlyserotonin.

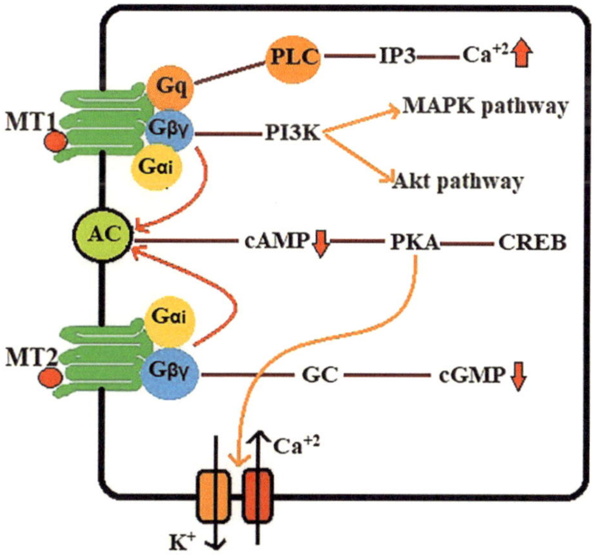

Figure 3.
MT 1 and MT 2 melatonin receptor signaling. PKA, protein kinase a; cAMP response element-binding protein; MT, melatonin receptor; Akt, threonine protein kinase B (PKB; also known as Akt); cyclic adenosine monophosphate; cGMP, cyclic guanosine monophosphate; CREB, IP3, inositol trisphosphate; MAPK, mitogen-activated protein kinase [18].

receptors and Gai/o proteins, it causes activity in the target tissue by regulating the levels of cAMP and calcium, the second messenger, as well as by regulating the activation of PKC subtypes (**Figure 3**) [19]. As a result of various studies, it has been determined that these receptors of Melatonin are in various structures of the brain belonging to the nervous system [20] as well as in nonneural tissues such as the immune system, endocrine system, bone, gastrointestinal system, cardiovascular system and reproductive organs, which we will focus on [21]. Again, as a result of a study, it was determined that melatonin causes various activities in various tissues through a mechanism independent of its receptors [22].

3. Melatonin receptors and their functions

It has been reported that melatonin synthesized by the pineal gland has 3 groups of receptors. These are MT1 receptors with high affinity. They are MT2 and MT3 receptors with low affinity [23–25]. MT1 stimulation from these receptors suppresses adenylate cyclase activity in the target tissue. It has been determined that these receptors are involved in retinal function, cerebral artery contraction, circadian rhythm, renal function, and reproduction. As a result of the stimulation of MT2 and MT3 receptors, phosphoinositol hydrolysis takes place in the target tissue [24, 25]. These receptors are located in the body of the brain, cardiovascular system, coronary and cerebral arteries, retina, ventricular wall, aorta, liver, and gall bladder, enterocytes, cecum, skin, colon, and appendix vermiformis, parotid gland, immune system cells, exocrine pancreas, kidney, platelets, ovary/granulosa cells, myometrium, placenta, and fetal kidney.

4. Effects of melatonin on the female reproductive system

Various studies have shown the effect of melatonin on the female reproductive system. It has been determined that this effect is by binding directly to the receptors in the cells in the ovary and through the hypothalamic/pituitary axis.

4.1 Direct effects of melatonin on the female reproductive system

Melatonin is considered to have an inhibitory effect on the hypothalamus-pituitary-gonads system. Demonstration of melatonin receptors in the ovary and structures such as mammary glands supports this effect. Studies have shown that melatonin receptors in rat ovarian tissue are more in the proestrus cycle than in the metestrus cycle and that granulosa cells are the main site for the MT1 receptor [26, 27]. The concentration of melatonin in follicular fluid was found to be ten times higher than in plasma. The source of the melatonin in the follicular fluid in circulation. The follicles receive this hormone from the bloodstream. The amount of hormone intake varies depending on the follicular growth period. The larger the follicles, the more melatonin is taken from the blood. Studies have reported that melatonin acts as an antioxidant in follicles and contributes to progesterone production by luteinizing granulosa cells [28]. Melatonin levels in humans during pregnancy and delivery are higher compared to the postpartum period [29]. Increased melatonin levels before birth may serve as an important circadian signal for the time of birth. Maternal melatonin originates from the maternal pineal gland and increases with the activities of placental hormones [28]. Melatonin, which is present in human follicular fluid in conjunction with plasma and does not affect granulosa cells' steroidogenesis and follicular function, directly affects ovarian function [30]. Periodic fluctuations are seen in the follicular fluid that fills the antral cavity, and there is more melatonin in the preovulatory follicle than in the serum level [31]. As a result of these findings, it is concluded that melatonin is synthesized in the ovary and released into the follicular fluid [32]. Studies have shown that LH receptors increase in granulosa cells as a result of melatonin administration [30]. Similarly, melatonin has been reported to affect sex steroid hormone production in follicular maturation during ovulation [33]. During follicular growth, locally produced insulin-like growth factors and transforming growth factor-β together with gonadotropins show efficacy [34]. In one study, it was reported that Melatonin stimulated the production of IGF-I in human granulosa cells [34]. Melatonin is also known to induce the IGFI receptor and activate the P13K/AKT signaling pathway, which is associated with cell metabolism, and the MEK/ERK signaling pathway, which is involved in cell growth, proliferation, and differentiation [35]. The TGF-β superfamily is found in ovarian cells and acts as an intraovarian regulator of follicle development [36]. As a result of studies, it has been determined that TGF-β is produced by both theca and granulosa cells in humans [37, 38]. Studies have shown that melatonin treatment increases TGF-β gene expression in mice [39]. Recent studies have shown that melatonin causes induction of Bcl2 expression and a decrease in Caspase-3 activity, thus protecting tissue from induction of the mitochondrial pathway of apoptosis [40]. The increase in follicular melatonin is an important factor for escaping from growing follicle deatresia, and the amount of intrafollicular melatonin is directly related to atresia [40]. It is stated that the increased amount of melatonin in the follicle may be associated with increased progesterone production after luteinization and ovulation. Local productions of ovarian progesterone, angiotensin-II, and nitric oxide synthetase (NOS) also increase with ovulation [41]. These vasoactive molecules have a fundamental role in the control of follicular blood flow [40]. An increase in progesterone and estradiol levels is required for successful ovulation [42]. Although there is no clear information about the relationship between melatonin, prostaglandin, and estradiol in anovulation, a study on rats showed that melatonin treatment in the gastric mucosa significantly increased the concentration of prostaglandin and estradiol [42]. ROS emerging in folliculogenesis suppresses the production of prostaglandin, which stimulates the synthesis of melatonin from granulosa cells, and induces corpus luteum transformation [43]. In addition to these properties, melatonin also protects the corpus luteum from damage by reactive oxygen species that inhibit progesterone production in human luteal cells.

4.2 Indirect effects of melatonin on the female reproductive system

Considering the indirect effects of melatonin on the female reproductive system. Melatonin exerts its indirect inhibitory effect on the gonads by suppressing the production and secretion of GnRH at the hypothalamus level, inhibiting the release of LH (Luteinizing hormone) from the pituitary, as well as suppressing LH secretion by acting directly on the pituitary by changing the levels of intracellular second messengers such as Ca^{2+} and cAMP. Melatonin also increases the secretion of opioid substances that reduce GnRH secretion, such as endorphins [44].

5. Effects of melatonin on the male reproductive system

Various studies have shown that melatonin has some effects on the male reproductive system as well as the female reproductive system. It has been determined that this effect is by binding to the receptors of Sertoli and Leydig cells in the testicles and via the hypothalamus/pituitary axis.

5.1 Direct effects of melatonin on the male reproductive system

When the direct effects of melatonin on testicular tissue are examined, it has been stated that melatonin affects testicular development by binding to the relevant receptors in the testis [45] and in a study, exogenous melatonin administration in rats caused a decrease in testicular size [46, 47]. Various studies have shown that MT1 and MT2 are expressed in the testes of young and adult rats [45]. In a study, it was observed that the external application of Melatonin had negative effects on the seminiferous tubules in the testicles of old male mice [48]. It has also been reported that the administration of melatonin causes shrinkage in testicular tissue and low spermatid count in rats [49]. In another study, significant morphological changes occurred in the tubular and interstitial compartments of the testicles in hamsters exposed to short-term sunlight for a long time [50]. In addition, it was determined that melatonin significantly reduced the volume of mitochondria and nongranular endoplasmic reticulum, which are organelles containing enzymes that have an important role in androgen biosynthesis in mice Leydig cells [51]. Looking at the mechanism of testosterone production, it was determined that the LH hormone released from the adenohypophysis stimulates the cAMP signal in Sertoli cells [52]. It was also stated that melatonin did not suppress the activity of P450scc and thus decreased steroid synthesis. It was determined that StAR protein expression regulated by melatonin LH or cAMP was significantly reduced [53]. Another pathway that is effective in the testosterone release mechanism is that GnRH does so by increasing cytosolic $Ca2+$ concentrations and activating protein kinase C [52]. In some studies using the fluorescent $Ca2+$ indicator, it has been reported that melatonin suppresses the release of GnRH-dependent $Ca2+$ from intracellular stores, thereby reducing cellular $Ca2+$ levels and suppressing testosterone release [54]. In addition to the aforementioned mechanisms, melatonin has been reported to regulate testosterone production by interacting with the CRH system in the testicles [55, 56]. It has been determined that the CRH hormone is produced in the testicles as well as the hypothalamus. CRH released from the testicles acts as an important negative autocrine regulator of LH-induced testosterone production [57]. In a study, it was reported that Melatonin administration significantly increased the levels of mRNA related to CRH in Leydig cells [58]. Another hormone involved in testicular function is Estrogen. In immature males, the main production site of estrogen is Sertoli cells. Estrogen receptor-alpha (ERα), one of the estrogen receptors, was found in Leydig cells, while ERβ, another estrogen receptor subtype, was found in Sertoli and germ cells [59, 60]. Studies show that ERβ plays a role in the regulation of Leydig cell proliferation and testosterone production in adult mouse testicles. The cytochrome P450 aromatase (P450arom) enzyme is a key enzyme found in the endoplasmic reticulum of various tissues and is responsible for the production of estrogen from androgens. P450arom enzyme has been identified in Leydig cells of several species [61]. Melatonin has been reported to reduce estrogen biosynthesis by inhibiting the activity and expression of aromatase [62–64]. It has been determined that the administration of melatonin in Leydig and Sertoli cells obtained from rams increases testosterone production by increasing the expression of stem cell factor and insulin-like growth factor-1 [65]. In addition, it was determined that melatonin administration regulated lactate metabolism in Sertoli cells. Lactate released from Sertoli cells provides nutritional support to cells and prevents apoptosis [66]. As a result of the studies, it has been determined that the level of melatonin in the semen is related to infertility [67–70]. Especially in rams, melatonin level is directly related to sperm quality. Although rams can produce semen throughout the year, the quality of sperm outside the breeding season has been found to be low [71]. In the studies, it was determined that the application of melatonin outside of the breeding season increased sperm volume in the semen [72–74]. It was also determined that the dividing ability of oocytes fertilized by spermatozoa treated with melatonin increased. This increase is mediated by the increase of hyaluronidase enzyme activity by the administration of melatonin [75, 76].

5.2 Indirect effects of melatonin on the male reproductive system

When the indirect effects of melatonin on the male reproductive system are examined, it has been determined that there is an effect, especially on the hypothalamus-pituitary axis. In a study, it was determined that the application of melatonin to the hypothalamus significantly reduced testicular weight [77–79]. It was concluded that it showed this effect by suppressing GnRH secretion. In another study, it was determined that the administration of melatonin to mice caused a decrease in testicular and seminal vesicle mass, thus causing a decrease in sperm count [80]. GnIH, a hormone that suppresses the release of GnRH, was determined in a study conducted on quails in 2000 [81–83]. It has been determined that the effect of melatonin on GnRH secretion is mediated by this hormone. It has been determined that melatonin stimulates the release of GnIH by binding to the MT1 receptor, thus suppressing the release of GnRH [84, 85]. It has been determined that melatonin hormone androgen receptor and ABP levels are decreased in animals with seasonal reproduction. In some animals, it has been determined that tonin has positive effects on the male reproductive system. For example, it has been determined that it has indirect effects as well as direct effects on rams. Melatonin administration has been found to increase the testosterone concentration of somatic cells in ram testis tissue [86, 87]. Kispeptins, which are stimulators of GnRH neurons, have been found to be highly effective in transmitting the melatonin message [88–90]. In a study, it was determined kisspeptin expression decreased and atrophy occurred in the gonaon in winter days when the daylight decreased in Syrian hamsters. It has been determined that the level of testosterone increases with the injection of kisspeptin [91, 92]. In a study with zebrafish, it was determined that melatonin administration could induce the expression of Kiss1 and Kiss2 and GnRH3 genes in brain tissue and an increase in LH-β in the pituitary gland [93]. This induced gonad development. However, in a study in rats, it was reported that the administration of melatonin suppressed the release of FSH and LH, thus suppressing spermatogenesis in Sertoli cells and delaying sexual maturation [94]. Again, it was determined that the administration of melatonin to rats in the fetal period suppressed LHRH release and significantly reduced the LH level [95, 96]. Melatonin administration is thought to inhibit LH release by reducing Ca^{2+} flow and cAMP concentrations in the pituitary gland [97].

6. The relationship between melatonin and oxidative stress

Oxidative stress is a cell-damaging condition that can result from decreased antioxidants and/or increased production of reactive free radicals such as reactive oxygen species and/or reactive nitrogen species (ROS/RSN) [98, 99]. Increased free radical production causes cell damage, leading to an increase in various damage markers (MDA, 8-OhDH, TNF-alpha) [100, 101]. In many cases, the body protects the cell against the increase in oxidative stress by the regulation of antioxidant defense systems

(GSH, SOD, CAT, GPx) [102–107]. If oxidative stress can be neutralized, there is usually no adverse contribution to disease pathology. If antioxidant defense induction is inadequate or absent, concomitant cellular and tissue damage often occurs. Some diseases can be directly caused by oxidative stress, but in most diseases, oxidative stress is a consequence and can often only be a secondary event [108–110]. However, it plays an important role in promoting additional tissue damage in most diseases. When oxidative stress is excessive, it can be prevented by using various substances that have antioxidant properties or suppressing oxidative stress to prevent cell damage [111, 112]. One of the substances used for this purpose is melatonin. As a result of various studies, it has been determined that melatonin reduces oxidative stress and protects the cell against oxidative damage. Some studies have stated that it prevents cell damage by improving MDA levels [113–116]. The effect of melatonin on reducing MDA occurs through several mechanisms. For example; Melatonin detoxifies a large number of free radicals such as peroxynitrite anion [117] and hydroxyl radical [118] detoxifies hydroxyl radical [119]. It has also been determined that peroxynitrous acid [120] cleans oxidizing particles such as nitric oxide [121] and thus prevents lipid peroxidation. Due to these effects, It has been reported that the effects of melatonin on oxidative stress are direct free radical scavenger and indirect antioxidant [122]. Again, as a result of studies, it was determined that Melatonin increased the level of antioxidant GSH, and also caused an increase in antioxidant enzyme activities such as GPX, SOD, and CAT. It has been determined that these effects are caused by an increase in mRNA expression by stimulating the melatonin receptors on the cell membrane [123]. It has also been determined that melatonin inhibits the nuclear translocation of NF-κB [124]. It has been determined that melatonin inhibits oxidative stress-induced DNA damage by suppressing oxidative stress [125]. Studies have shown that melatonin inhibits apoptosis by decreasing caspase-3 activity and activating the PI3K/AKT pathway, and it preserves membrane integrity. Activation of the PI3K/AKT pathway also increases gene expression such as Nrf2 [126], which plays an important role in the antioxidant defense system. These findings explain the cell-protective mechanism of melatonin against oxidative stress.

7. Conclusion

Melatonin is a hormone mainly synthesized from the pineal gland, and it has been shown by some studies that it has various effects on the immune system, oxidative stress, and reproduction, as well as taking part in the regulation of circadian rhythm. In this study, we focused on the direct, indirect, and antioxidant effects of melatonin on the female and male reproductive systems and the molecular mechanisms of these effects. As a result, melatonin affects the male and female reproductive systems directly via the gonads via secondary messengers and indirectly by stimulating various receptors/molecules via the hypothalamus-pituitary axis. These effects are in the direction of supporting reproduction in some living things and suppressing in others. In addition, melatonin prevents cell damage by increasing antioxidant enzyme activity and scavenging free radicals, especially in female and male gonads, thus preventing cell damage.

Author details

Volkan Gelen[1*], Emin Şengül[2] and Abdulsamed Kükürt[3]

1 Faculty of Veterinary Medicine, Department of Physiology, Kafkas University, Kars, Turkey

2 Faculty of Veterinary Medicine, Department of Physiology, Atatürk University, Erzurum, Turkey

3 Faculty of Veterinary Medicine, Department of Biochemistry, Kafkas University, Kars, Turkey

*Address all correspondence to: gelen_volkan@hotmail.com

References

[1] Cipolla-Neto J, Amaral FGD. Melatonin as a hormone: New physiological and clinical insights. Endocrine Reviews. 2018;**39**(6):990-1028

[2] Pevet P. Melatonin. Dialogues in Clinical Neuroscience. 2002;**4**(1):57-72

[3] Pevet P, Challet E. Melatonin: Both master clock output and internal time-giver in the circadian clocks network. Journal of Physiology, Paris. 2011;**105**(4-6):170-182

[4] Bubenik GA. Gastrointestinal melatonin: Localization, function, and clinical relevance. Digestive Diseases and Sciences. 2002;**47**:2336-2348

[5] Slominski A, Fischer TW, Zmijewski MA, Wortsman J, Semak I, Zbytek B, et al. On the role of melatonin in skin physiology and pathology. Endocrine. 2005;**27**:137-148

[6] Carrillo-Vico A, Calvo JR, Abreu P, Lardone PJ, GarcíaMauriño S, Reiter RJ, et al. Evidence of melatonin synthesis by human lymphocytes and its physiological significance: Possible role as intracrine, autocrine, and/or paracrine substance. The FASEB Journal. 2004;**18**:537-539

[7] Cardinali DP, Rosner JM. Metabolism of serotonin by the rat retina in vitro. Journal of Neurochemistry. 1971;**18**:1769-1770

[8] Berson DM, Dunn FA, Takao M. Phototransduction by retinal ganglion cells that set the circadian clock. Science. 2002;**295**:1070-1073. DOI: 10.1126/science.1067262

[9] Simoneaux V, Ribelayga C. Generation of the melatonin endocrine message in mammals: A review of the complex regulation of melatonin synthesis by norepinephrine, peptides, and other pineal transmitters. Pharmacological Reviews. 2003;**55**(2):325-395

[10] Ölmez E, Şahna E, Ağkadir M, Acet A. Melatonin: emeklilik yaşı 80 olur mu? Turgut Özal Tıp Dergisi. 2000;**7**:177-187

[11] Sack RL, Lewy AJ, Hughes RJ. Use of melatonin for sleep and circadian rhythm disorders. Annals of Medicine. 1998;**30**:115-121

[12] Çam A, Erdoğan MF. Melatonin. Ankara Üniversitesi Tıp Fakültesi. Mecmuası. 2003;**56**:103-112

[13] Cipolla-Neto J, Amaral FG, Soares JM Jr, Gallo CC, Furtado A, Cavaco JE, et al. The crosstalk between melatonin and sex steroid hormones. Neuroendocrinology. 2022;**112**(2):115-129

[14] Skwarlo-Sonta K, Majewski P, Markowska M, Oblap R, Olszanska B. Bidirectional communication between the pineal gland and the imimune system. Canadian Journal of Physiology and Pharmacology. 2003;**81**(4):342-349

[15] Mayo JC, Aguado A, Cernuda-Cernuda R, Álvarez-Artime A, Cepas V, Quirós-González I, et al. Melatonin uptake by cells: an answer to its relationship with glucose? Molecules. 10 Aug 2018;**23**(8):1999

[16] Amaral FGD, Cipolla-Neto J. A brief review about melatonin, a pineal hormone. Archives of Endocrinology and Metabolism. 2018;**62**(4):472-479

[17] Liu J, Clough SJ, Hutchinson AJ, AdamahBiassi EB, Popovska-Gorevski M, Dubocovich ML. MT1 and MT2

melatonin receptors: A therapeutic perspective. Annual Review of Pharmacology and Toxicology. 2016;**56**:361-383

[18] Masana MI, Dubocovich ML. Melatonin receptor signaling: finding the path through the dark. Science STKE. 2001;**6**(107):39

[19] Pandi-Perumal SR, Trakht I, Srinivasan V, Spence DW, Maestroni GJ, Zisapel N, et al. Physiological effects of melatonin: Role of melatonin receptors and signal transduction pathways. Progress in Neurobiology. 2008;**85**(3):335-353

[20] Ng KY, Leong MK, Liang H, Paxinos G. Melatonin receptors: Distribution in the mammalian brain and their respective putative functions. Brain Structure & Function. 2017;**222**(7):2921-2939

[21] Slominski RM, Reiter RJ, Schlabritz-Loutsevitch N, Ostrom RS, Slominski AT. Melatonin membrane receptors in peripheral tissues: Distribution and functions. Molecular and Cellular Endocrinology. 2012;**351**(2):152-166

[22] Reiter RJ, Tan DX, Galano A. Melatonin: Exceedance meditations. Physiology. 2014;**29**(5):325-333

[23] Conway S, Canning SJ, Howell HE, Mowat ES, Barrett P, Drew JE, et al. Characterisation of human melatonin mt(1) and MT(2) receptors by CRE-luciferase reporter assay. European Journal of Pharmacology. 2000;**390**:15-24

[24] Pintor J, Martin L, Pelaez T, Hoyle CH, Peral A. Involvement of melatonin MT(3) receptors in the regulation of intraocular pressure in rabbits. European Journal of Pharmacology. 2001;**416**:251-254

[25] Grosjean O, Ferro M, Coge F, Beauverger P, Henlin JM, Lefoulon F, et al. Identification of the melatonin binding site MT3 as the quinone reductase 2. The Journal of Biological Chemistry. 2000;**275**:31311-31317

[26] Conway S, Canning SJ, Howell HE, Mowat ES, Barrett P, Drew JE, et al. Characterisation of human melatonin mt(1) and MT(2) receptors by CRE-luciferase reporter assay. European Journal of Pharmacology. 2000;**390**:15-24

[27] Pintor J, Martin L, Pelaez T, Hoyle CH, Peral A. Involvement of melatonin MT(3) receptors in the regulation of intraocular pressure in rabbits. European Journal of Pharmacology. 2001;**416**:251-254

[28] Şahin D. İn vitro koşullarda sirkadien melatonin etkisine maruz bırakılan embriyolarda SOD ve HMGB1 genlerinin ekspresyonları ile melatonin etkisinin takibi. istanbul: istanbul Bilim Üniversitesi; 2014

[29] Wierrani F, Grin W, Hlawka B, Kroiss A, Grünberger W. Elevated serum melatonin levels during human late pregnancy and labour. Journal of Obstetrics and Gynaecology. 1997;**17**:449-451

[30] Woo MMM, Tai CJ, Kang SK, et al. Direct action of melatonin in human granulosa-luteal cells. The Journal of Clinical Endocrinology and Metabolism. 2001;**86**:4789-4797

[31] Maitra SK, Chattoraj A, Mukherjee S, et al. Melatonin: A potent candidate in the regulation of fish oocyte growth and maturation. General and Comparative Endocrinology. 2013;**181**:215-222

[32] Sakaguchi K, Itoh MT, Takahashi N, et al. The rat oocyte synthesizes melatonin. Reproduction, Fertility, and Development. 2013;**25**:674-682

[33] Danforth DR. Endocrine and paracrine control of oocyte development. American Journal of Obstetrics & Gynecology. 1995;**172**:747-752

[34] Poretsky L, Cataldo NA, Rosenwaks Z, et al. The insulin-related ovarian regülatöry system in health and disease. Endocrinology Reviews. 1999;**20**:535-582

[35] Chun SY, Billig H, Tilly JL, et al. Gonadotropin suppression of apoptosis in cultured preovulatory follicles: Mediatory role of endogenous insulin-like growth factor I. Endocrinology. 1994;**135**:1845-1853

[36] Tilly JL. Tilly KI inhibitors of oxidative stress mimic the ability of follicle- stimulating hormone to suppress apoptosis in cultured rat ovarian follicles. Endocrinology. 1995;**136**:242-252

[37] Knight PG, Glister C. TGF-beta süper family members and ovarian follicle development. Reproduction. 2006;**132**:191-206

[38] Tatemoto H, Muto N, Sunagawa I, et al. Protection of porcine oocytes against cell damage caused by oxidative stress during In vitro maturation: Role of superoxide dismutase activity in porcine follicular fluid. Biology of Reproduction. 2004;**71**:1150-1157

[39] Ratts VS, Flaws JA, Kolp R, et al. Ablation of bcl-2 gene expression decreases the numbers of oocyte sand primordial follicles established in the post-natal female mouse gonad. Endocrinology. 1995;**136**:3665-3668

[40] Tamura H, Takasaki A, Ichiro M, et al. Oxidative stress impairs oocyte quality and melatonin protects oocytes from free radical damage and improves fertilization rate. Journal of Pineal Research. 2008;**44**:280-287

[41] Matikainen T, Perez GI, Zheng TS, et al. Caspase-3 gene knockout defines cell lineage specificity for programmed cell death signaling in the ovary. Endocrinology. 2001;**142**:2468-2480

[42] Nakamura Y, Tamura H, Takayama H, et al. Increased endogenous level of melatonin in preovulatory human follicles does not directly influence progesterone production. Fertility and Sterility. 2003;**80**:1012-1016

[43] Wetterberg L, Arendt J, Paunier L, et al. Human serum melatonin changes during the menstrual cycle. The Journal of Clinical Endocrinology and Metabolism. 1976;**42**:185-188

[44] Aleandri V, Spina V, Morini A. The pineal gland and reproduction. Human Reproduction Update. 1996;**2**:225-223

[45] Izzo G, Francesco A, Ferrara D, et al. Expression of melatonin (MT1, MT2) and melatonin-related receptors in the adult rat testes and during development. Zygote. 2010;**18**:257-264

[46] Edmonds KE, StetsonMH. Photoperiod and melatonin affect testicular growth in the marsh rice rat (Oryzomys palustris). Journal of Pineal Research. 1994;**17**:86-93

[47] Edmonds KE, Stetson MH. Pineal gland and melatonin affect testicular status in the adult marsh rice rat (Oryzomys palustris). General and Comparative Endocrinology. 1995;**99**:265-274

[48] Mehraein F, Negahdar F. Morphometric evaluation of

seminiferous tubules in aged mice testes after melatonin administration. Cell Journal. 2011;**13**:1-4

[49] Rashed RA, Mohamed IK, Ei-Alfy SH. Effects of two different doses of melatonin on the spermatogenic cells of rat testes: A light and electron microscopic study. Egypt Journal of Histology. 2010;**33**:819-835

[50] Mason AO, Duffy S, Zhao S, et al. Photoperiod and reproductive condition are associated with changes in RFamide-related peptide (RFRP) expression in Syrian hamsters (Mesocricetus auratus). Journal of Biological Rhythms. 2010;**25**:176-185

[51] Redins CA, Redins GM, Novaes JC. The effects of treatment with melatonin on the ultrastructure ofmouse Leydig cells: A quantitative study. Brazilian Journal of Biology. 2002;**62**:517-523

[52] Stojilković SS, Chang JP, Ngo D, Tasaka K, Izumi S, Catt KJ. Mechanism of action of GnRH: The participation of calcium mobilization and activation of protein kinase C in gonadotropin secretion. Journal of Steroid Biochemistry. 1989;**33**:693-703

[53] Wu CS, Leu SF, Yang HY, Huang BM. Melatonin inhibits the expression of steroidogenic acute regulatory protein and steroidogenesis in MA-10 cells. Journal of Andrology. 2001;**22**:245-254

[54] Valenti S, Thellung S, Florio T, Giusti M, Schettini G, Giordano G. A novel mechanism for the melatonin inhibition of testosterone secretion by rat Leydig cells: Reduction of GnRH-induced increase in cytosolic Ca2+. Journal of Molecular Endocrinology. 1999;**23**:299-306

[55] Frungieri MB, Mayerhofer A, Zitta K, Pignataro OP, Calandra RS, Gonzalez-Calvar SI. Direct effect ofmelatonin on Syrian hamster testes: Melatonin subtype 1a receptors, inhibition of androgen production, and interaction with the local corticotropinreleasing hormone system. Endocrinology. 2005;**146**:1541-1552

[56] Yao M, Schulkin J, Denver RJ. Evolutionarily conserved glucocorticoid regulation of corticotropin-releasing factor expression. Endocrinology. 2008;**149**:2352-2360

[57] Dufau ML, Tinajero JC, Fabbri A. Corticotropin-releasing factor: An antireproductive hormone of the testis. The FASEB Journal. 1993;7:299-307

[58] Rossi SP, Matzkin ME, Terradas C, et al. New insights into melatonin/CRH signaling in hamster Leydig cells. General and Comparative Endocrinology. 2012;**178**:153-163

[59] Bili ′ nska B, Schmalz-Fraczek B, Kotula M, Carreau S. Photoperiod-dependent capability of androgen aromatization and the role of estrogens in the bank vole testis visualized by means of immunohistochemistry. Molecular and Cellular Endocrinology. 2001;**178**:189-198

[60] Gould ML, Hurst PR, Nichol HD. The effects of oestrogen receptors alpha and beta on testicular cell number and steroidogenesis in mice. Reproduction. 2007;**134**:271-279

[61] Carreau S. Germ cells: A new source of estrogens in the male gonad. Molecular and Cellular Endocrinology. 2001;**178**:65-72

[62] Letellier K, Azeddine B, Parent S, Labelle H, Rompré PH, Moreau A, et al. Estrogen cross-talk with the melatonin signaling pathway in human osteoblasts derived from adolescent idiopathic

scoliosis patients. Journal of Pineal Research. 2008;**45**:383-393

[63] Yoshitane H, Honma S, Imamura K, Nakajima H, Nishide SY, Ono D, et al. JNK regulates the photic response of the mammalian circadian clock. EMBO Reports. 2012;**13**:455-461

[64] Vriend J, Reiter RJ. Breast cancer: Modulation by melatonin and the ubiquitin-proteasome system–a review. Molecular and Cellular Endocrinology. 2015;**417**:1-9. [Cross Ref] [PubMed]

[65] Deng SL, Wang ZP, Jin C, Kang XL, Batool A, Zhang Y, et al. Melatonin promotes sheep Leydig cell testosterone secretion in a co-culture with Sertoli cells. Theriogenology. 2018;**106**:170-177

[66] Rocha CS, Martins AD, Rato L, Silva BM, Oliveira PF, Alves MG. Melatonin alters the glycolytic profile of Sertoli cells: Implications for male fertility. Molecular Human Reproduction. 2014;**20**:1067-1076

[67] Awad H, Halawa F, Mostafa T, Atta H. Melatonin hormone profile in infertile males. International Journal of Andrology. 2006;**29**:409-413

[68] Yie SM, Daya S, Brown GM, Deys L, YoungLai EV. Melatonin and aromatase stimulating activity of human seminal plasma. Andrologia. 1999;**23**:227-231

[69] van Vuuren RJ, Pitout MJ, van Aswegen CH, Theron JJ. Putativemelatonin receptor in human spermatozoa. Clinical Biochemistry. 1992;**25**:125-127

[70] Casao A, Gallego M, Abecia JA, et al. Identification and immunolocalisation of melatonin MT(1) and MT(2) receptors in rasa Aragonesa ram spermatozoa. Reproduction, Fertility, and Development. 2012;**24**:953-961

[71] Azawi OI, Al-Khashab ANTM, Al-Kadoo NN. Effect of gonadotropin releasing hormone treatment on semen characteristics and enzymatic activities of Awassi rams in breeding and non-breeding seasons. Iranian Journal of Applied Animal Science. 2012;**2**:13-19

[72] Ramadan TA, Taha TA, Samak MA, Hassan A. Effectiveness of exposure to longday followed by melatonin treatment on semen characteristics of Damascus male goats during breeding and non-breeding seasons. Theriogenology. 2009;**71**:458-468

[73] Casao A, Vega S, Palacín I, et al. Effects of melatonin implants during non-breeding season on sperm motility and reproductive parameters in rasa Aragonesa rams. Reproduction in Domestic Animals. 2010;**45**:425-432

[74] Casao A, Mendoza N, Pérez-Pé R, et al. Melatonin prevents capacitation and apoptotic-like changes of ram spermatozoa and increases fertility rate. Journal of Pineal Research. 2010;**48**:39-46

[75] Tanyiladizi S, Bozkurt T, ÇİftÇİ O, SAKİN F. In vitro effects ofmelatonin on hyaluronidase activity and sperm motility in bull semen. Turk J vet. Animal Science. 2006;**30**:89-93

[76] Luboshitzky R, Shen-Orr Z, Nave R, Lavi S, Lavie P. Melatonin administration alters semen quality in healthy men. Journal of Andrology. 2002;**23**:572-578

[77] Wierman ME, Bruder JM, Kepa JK. Regulation of gonadotropin-releasing hormone (GnRH) gene expression in hypothalamic neuronal cells. Cellular and Molecular Neurobiology. 1995;**15**:79-88

[78] Weaver DR, Stehle JH, Stopa EG, Reppert SM. Melatonin receptors in human hypothalamus and pituitary:

Implications for circadian and reproductive responses to melatonin. The Journal of Clinical Endocrinology and Metabolism. 1993;**76**:295-301

[79] Glass JD, Knotts LK. A brain site for the antigonadal action of melatonin in the whitefooted mouse (Peromyscus leucopus): Involvement of the immunoreactive GnRH neuronal system. Neuroendocrinology. 1987;**46**:48-55

[80] Forger NG, Zucker I. Photoperiodic regulation of reproductive development in male white-footed mice (Peromyscus leucopus) born at different phases of the breeding season. Journal of Reproduction and Fertility. 1985;**73**:271-278

[81] Tsutsui K, Saigoh E, Ukena K, et al. A novel avian hypothalamic peptide inhibiting gonadotropin release. Biochemical and Biophysical Research Communications. 2000;**275**:661-667

[82] Ubuka T, Son YL, Bentley GE, Millar RP, Tsutsui K. Gonadotropin-inhibitory hormone (GnIH), GnIH receptor and cell signaling. General and Comparative Endocrinology. 2013;**190**:10-17

[83] Tsutsui K, Ubuka T, Bentley GE, Kriegsfeld LJ. Review: Regulatory mechanisms of gonadotropin-inhibitory hormone (GnIH) synthesis and release in photoperiodic animals. Frontiers in Neuroscience. 2013;7:60

[84] Tsutsui K, Ubuka T, Yin H, et al. Mode of action and functional significance of avian gonadotropin-inhibitory hormone (GnIH): A review. Journal of Experimental Zoology. Part A, Comparative Experimental Biology. 2006;**305**:801-806

[85] Reiter RJ, Tan DX, Rosales-Corral S, Manchester LC. The universal nature, unequal distribution and antioxidant functions of melatonin and its derivatives. Mini Reviews in Medicinal Chemistry. 2013;**13**:373-384

[86] Viguie C, Caraty A, Locatelli A, Malpaux B. Regulation of luteinizing hormone-releasing hormone (LHRH) secretion by melatonin in the ewe. II. Changes in N-methyl-DL-aspartic acid-induced LHRH release during the stimulation of luteinizing hormone secretion by melatonin. Biology of Reproduction. 1995;**52**:1156-1161

[87] Deng SL, Chen SR, Wang ZP, Zhang Y, Tang JX, Li J, et al. Melatonin promotes development of haploid germ cells from early developing spermatogenic cells of Suffolk sheep under in vitro condition. Journal of Pineal Research. 2016;**60**:435-447

[88] Buchanan KL, Yellon SM. Delayed puberty in the male Djungarian hamster: Effect of short photoperiod or melatonin treatment on the GnRH neuronal system. Neuroendocrinology. 1991;**54**:96-102

[89] Ancel C, Bentsen AH, Sébert ME, Tena-Sempere M, Mikkelsen JD, Simonneaux V. Stimulatory effect of RFRP-3 on the gonadotrophic axis in the male Syrian hamster: The exception proves the rule. Endocrinology. 2012;**153**:1352-1363

[90] Irwig MS, Fraley GS, Smith JT, Acohido BV, Popa SM, Cunningham MJ, et al. Kisspeptin activation of gonadotropin releasing hormone neurons and regulation of KiSS-1 mRNA in the male rat. Neuroendocrinology. 2004;**80**:264-272

[91] Ansel L, Bentsen AH, Ancel C, Bolborea M, Klosen P, Mikkelsen JD, et al. Peripheral kisspeptin reverses short photoperiod-induced gonadal regression in Syrian hamsters by promoting GNRH release. Reproduction. 2011;**142**:417-425

[92] Henningsen JB, Poirel VJ, Mikkelsen JD, Tsutsui K, Simonneaux V, Gauer F. Sex differences in the photoperiodic regulation of RF-amide related peptide (RFRP) and its receptor GPR147 in the Syrian hamster. The Journal of Comparative Neurology. 2016;**524**:1825-1838

[93] Carnevali O, Gioacchini G, Maradonna F, Olivotto I, Migliarini B. Melatonin induces follicle maturation in Danio rerio. PLoS One. 2011;**6**:e19978

[94] Lang U, Aubert ML, Rivest RW, Vinas-Bradtke JC, Sizonenko PC. Daily afternoon administration of melatonin does not irreversibly inhibit sexual maturation in the male rat. Endocrinology. 1984;**115**:2303-2310

[95] Martin JE, Sattler C. Selectivity of melatonin pituitary inhibition for luteinizing hormone-releasing hormone. Neuroendocrinology. 1982;**34**:112-116

[96] Hattori A, Herbert DC, Vaughan MK, Yaga K, Reiter RJ. Melatonin inhibits luteinizing hormone releasing hormone (LHRH) induction of LH release from fetal rat pituitary cells. Neuroscience Letters. 1995;**184**:109-112

[97] Vanecek J. Melatonin inhibits release of luteinizing hormone (LH) via decrease of [Ca2+] and cyclic AMP. Physiological Research. 1998;**47**:329-335

[98] Kükürt A, Gelen V, Başer ÖF, Deveci HA, Karapehlivan M. Thiols: Role in oxidative stress-related disorders. In: Lipid Peroxidation [Working Title]. London, UK: IntechOpen; 2021. DOI: 10.5772/intechopen.96682

[99] Kara A, Gedikli S, Sengul E, Gelen V, Ozkanlar S. Oxidative Stress and Autophagy. 1st ed. London: InTechOpen, Free Radicals and Diseases; 2016. pp. 69-86

[100] Gelen V, Yıldırım S, Şengül E, Çınar A, Çelebi F, Küçükkalem M, et al. Naringin attenuates oxidative stress, inflammation, apoptosis, and oxidative DNA damage in acrylamide-induced nephrotoxicity in rats. Asian Pacific Journal of Tropical Biomedicine. 2022;**12**(5):223-232

[101] Gelen V, Şengül E, Yıldırım S, Atila G. The protective effects of naringin against 5-fluorouracil-induced hepatotoxicity and nephrotoxicity in rats. Iranian Journal of Basic Medical Sciences. 2018;**21**(4):404-410. DOI: 10.22038/IJBMS.2018.27510.6714

[102] Karamese M, Guvendi B, Karamese SA, Cinar I, Can S, Erol HS, et al. The protective effects of epigallocatechin gallate on lipopolysaccharide-induced hepatotoxicity: An in vitro study on Hep3B cells. Iranian Journal of Basic Medical Sciences. 2016;**19**:483-489

[103] Gelen V, Sengul E. Antioxidant, anti-inflammatory, and antiapoptotic effects of naringin on cardiac damage induced by cisplatin. IJTK. 2020;**19**(2):459-465

[104] Sengul E, Gelen V, Yildirim S, et al. The effects of selenium in acrylamide-induced nephrotoxicity in rats: Roles of oxidative stress, inflammation, apoptosis, and DNA damage. Biological Trace Element Research. 2021;**199**:173-184

[105] Şengül E, Gelen V, Gedikli S, Özkanlar S, Gür G, Çelebi F. The protective effect of quercetin on cyclophosphamide-induced lung toxicity in rats. Biomedicine & Pharmacotherapy. 2017;**92**:303-307

[106] Sengul E, Gelen V, Gedikli S. Cardioprotective activities of quercetin and Rutin in Sprague Dawley rats treated

with 5-fluorouracil. Journal of Animal and Plant Sciences. 2021;**31**(2):423-431

[107] Kükürt A, Karapehlivan M. Protective effect of astaxanthin on experimental ovarian damage in rats. Journal of Biochemical and Molecular Toxicology. 2022;**36**(3):e22966. DOI: 10.1002/jbt.22966

[108] Gelen V, Kükürt A, Şengül E, Devecı HA. Leptin and its role in oxidative stress and apoptosis: An overview. In: Role of Obesity in Human Health and Disease. [Working Title],. London, UK: IntechOpen; 2021. DOI: 10.5772/intechopen.101237

[109] Gelen V, Kükürt A, Şengül E, Başer ÖF, Karapehlivan M. Can polyphenols be used as anti-inflammatory agents against Covid-19 (SARS-CoV-2)- induced inflammation? In: Badria FA, editor. Phenolic Compd. [Working Title]. Rijeka: IntechOpen; 2021. pp. 1-21. DOI: 10.5772/intechopen.98684

[110] Gelen V, Kükürt A, Şengül E. Role of the renin-angiotensin-aldosterone system in various disease processes: An overview. In: Renin-Angiotensin Aldosterone Syst. [Working Title]. London, UK: IntechOpen; 2021. DOI: 10.5772/intechopen.97354

[111] Gelen V, Şengül E, Yıldırım S, Senturk E, Tekin S, Kükürt A. The protective effects of hesperidin and curcumin on 5-fluorouracil–induced nephrotoxicity in mice. Environmental Science and Pollution Research. 2021. DOI: 10.1007/s11356-021-13969-5

[112] Gedikli S, Ozkanlar S, Gur C, Sengul E, Gelen V. Preventive effects of quercetin on liver damages in high-fat diet-induced obesity. Journal of Histology & Histopathology. 2017;**4**:7. DOI: 10.7243/2055-091X-4-7

[113] Fulia F, Gitto E, Cuzzocrea S, Reiter RJ, Dugo L, Gitto P, et al. Increased levels of malondialdehyde and nitrite/nitrate in the blood of asphyxiated newborns: Reduction by melatonin. Journal of Pineal Research. 2001;**31**(4):343-349

[114] Allegra M, Gentile C, Tesoriere L, Livrea M. Protective effect of melatonin against cytotoxic actions of malondialdehyde: An in vitro study on human erythrocytes. Journal of Pineal Research. 2002;**32**(3):187-193

[115] Ziaadini F, Aminae M, Rastegar MM, Abbasian S, Memari AH. Melatonin supplementation decreases aerobic exercise training induced-lipid peroxidation and malondialdehyde in sedentary young women. Polish Journal of Food and Nutrition Sciences. 2017;**67**(3):225-232

[116] Gedikli S, Gelen V, Sengul E, Ozkanlar S, Gur C, Agırbas O, et al. Therapeutic effects of melatonin on liver and kidney damages In intensive exercise model of rats. Endocrine, Metabolic & Immune Disorders Drug Targets. 2015;**15**(4):308-314

[117] Karbownik M, Reiter RJ. Antioxidative effects of melatonin in protection against cellular damage caused by ionizing radiation. Proceedings of the Society for Experimental Biology and Medicine. 2000;**22**:9-22

[118] Goc Z, Szaroma W, Kapusta E, Dziubek K. Protective effects of melatonin on the activity of SOD, CAT, GSH-Px and GSH content in organs of mice after administration of SNP. The Chinese Journal of Physiology. 2017;**60**(1):1-10

[119] Purushothaman A, Sheeja AA, Janardanan D. Hydroxyl radical scavenging activity of melatonin

and its related indolamines, Free Radicals. Res. 2020;**54**(5):373-383

[120] Loren P, Sanchez R, Arias ME, Felmer R, Risopatron J, Cheuqueman C. Melatonin scavenger properties against oxidative and nitrosative stress: Impact on gamete handling and in vitro embryo production in humans and other mammals. International Journal of Molecular Sciences. 2017;**18**(6):1119

[121] Fan W, He Y, Guan X, Gu W, Wu Z, Zhu X. el al, Involvement of the nitric oxide in melatonin-mediated protection against injury. Life Sciences. 2018;**200**:142-147

[122] Reina M, Martínez A. A new free radical scavenging cascade involving melatonin and three of its metabolites (3OHM, AFMK and AMK). Computational & Theoretical Chemistry. 2018;**1123**:111-118

[123] Ghosh AK, Naaz S, Bhattacharjee B, Ghosal N, Chattopadhyay A, Roy S, et al. Mechanism of melatonin protection against copperascorbate-induced oxidative damage in vitro through isothermal titration calorimetry. Life Sciences. 2017;**180**:123-136

[124] Dehghani S, Hosseini M, Haghgoo S, Changizi V, Akbari Javar H, Khoobi M, et al. Multifunctional MIL-Cur@ FC as a theranostic agent for magnetic resonance imaging and targeting drug delivery: in vitro and in vivo study. Journal of Drug Targeting. 2020;**28**(6):668-680

[125] Okatani Y, Wakatsuki A, Shinohara K, Kaneda C, Fukaya T. Melatonin stimulates glutathione peroxidase activity in human chorion. Journal of Pineal Research. 2001;**30**(4):199-205

[126] Zhang Y, Wei Z, Liu W, Wang J, He X, Huang H, et al. Melatonin protects against arsenic trioxide-induced liver injury by the upregulation of Nrf2 expression through the activation of PI3K/AKT pathway. Oncotarget. 2017;**8**(3):3773

Section 3

The Antioxidant Effect of Melatonin

Chapter 3

Biochemistry and Antioxidant Effects of Melatonin

Oguz Merhan

Abstract

Melatonin (N-acetyl-5-methoxy-tryptamine) is a hormone taking place in many biological and physiological processes, such as reproduction, sleep, antioxidant effect, and circadian rhythm (biological clock), and is a multifunctional indolamine compound synthesized mainly from the metabolism of tryptophan via serotonin in the pineal gland. Melatonin, which is a hormone synthesized from the essential amino acid tryptophan, is substantially secreted from the pineal gland between the cerebral hemispheres found in the mammalian brain. In addition to this, it is also produced in the cells and tissues, such as the gastrointestinal system, gall, epithelial hair follicles, skin, retina, spleen, testis, salivary glands, bone marrow, leukocytes, placenta, and thrombocytes. It plays a role in many physiological events, such as synchronizing circadian rhythms, reproduction, fattening, molting, hibernation, and change of pigment granules, preserving the integrity of the gastrointestinal system with an anti-ulcerative effect in tissues and organs from which it is produced. Melatonin is also a powerful antioxidant and anti-apoptotic agent that prevents oxidative and nitrosative damage to all macromolecules due to its ability to form in metabolic activities, directly excrete toxic oxygen derivatives, and reduce the formation of reactive oxygen and nitrogen species. In this book chapter, we will explain the structure, synthesis, metabolism, and antioxidant effects of the melatonin hormone.

Keywords: antioxidant, biochemistry, melatonin, shikimate pathway, tryptophan

1. Introduction

Melatonin (N-acetyl-5-methoxy-tryptamine) is a hormone taking place in many biological and physiological processes and is a multifunctional indolamine compound synthesized mainly from the metabolism of tryptophan via serotonin in the pineal gland [1]. Its molecular formula is $C_{13}H_{16}N_2O_2$ and its molecular weight is 232.278 g/mol (**Figure 1**) [2]. It has the capacity to be able to pass through all biological membranes due to its small molecular size and high lipophilicity and it is evenly distributed to all biological tissues and fluids by crossing the blood–brain barrier [3].

Although the existence of the pineal gland has been known since ancient times, the French philosopher Rene Descartes described the pineal gland as the "throne of the soul" about three hundred years ago [4]. Melatonin hormone was first described in 1958 by the American dermatologist Aaron Lerner by obtaining from the pineal gland of cattle [5]. Melatonin, which is produced in the cells called pinealocytes of

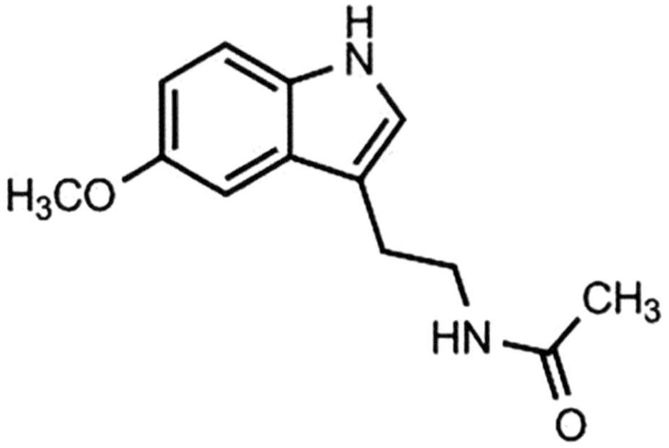

Figure 1.
Chemical structure of melatonin.

the pineal gland, is a hormone that plays a role in the regulation of many physiological and biological functions, such as circadian rhythm, sleep/wake cycle, pubertal development-reproduction, locomotor activity, regulation of immunity and blood pressure, molting, and hibernation [6–10].

Cortisol and melatonin levels act in opposite directions. Immediately after cortisol levels drop at night, melatonin levels begin to increase. The balance between these two hormones is important for good health and various diseases can occur with low melatonin and high cortisol levels [11, 12].

While melatonin shows a stimulating effect on the gonads in animals, such as sheep, goats, and deer, it shows suppressive properties in animals, such as horses, hamsters, and camels [13]. Melatonin acts as a timer by providing to follow-up the changes in the light/dark ratio of the animal seasonally [14].

In sheep, melatonin secretion and plasma levels are low in daylight [15, 16]. After sunset, melatonin secretion increases 10–20 times and rises rapidly to reach a peak by the end of the night. Thus, melatonin signal reflects the duration of the dark phase [14]. Melatonin initiates a series of events that lead to the start of the reproduction season [17]. The decreasing light exposure time increases melatonin secretion in the autumn-winter months when the days start to get shorter. Increased melatonin secretion stimulates gonadotrophin-releasing hormone (GnRH) secretion and provides to initiate estrus by acting on the hypothalamus in sheep [18, 19].

2. Melatonin

2.1 Tryptophan synthesis

The shikimate pathway is found in bacteria, fungi, plants, and algae, as well as in some protozoans. However, this pathway does not occur in animals and therefore animals must obtain aromatic amino acids from their diets as essential nutrients. Phosphoenolpyruvate (PEP), sugar with 3-carbon, product of the glycolysis pathway and erythrose-4-phosphate (E4-P), sugar with 4-carbon, synthesized from the pentose phosphate pathway starts with its conversion to

2-keto-3-deoxy-D-arabinoheptulosonate 7-phosphate, 7-carbon compound, with the hydrolysis of phosphate by 2-keto-3-deoxy-D-arabino-heptulosonate 7-phosphate synthase enzyme [20, 21].

In the second reaction, 3-dehydroquinate, a cyclic product, occurs by elimination of phosphate from 2-keto-3-deoxy-D-arabinoheptulosonate 7-phosphate by the catalysis of 3-dehydroquinate synthase enzyme with the help of NAD^+. 3-dehydroshikimate is formed from this product with the effect of 3-dehydroquinate dehydratase enzyme as a result of the loss of the H_2O molecule [20, 22].

The next reaction is the reduction of 3-dehydroshikimate to shikimate by the shikimate dehydrogenase enzyme, which is used as a cofactor with NADPH. It is converted to shikimate 3-phosphate by the shikimate kinase enzyme by using one ATP per molecule. 5-enolpyruvylshikimate-3-phosphate is formed from shikimate 3-phosphate by binding to phosphoenolpyruvate (PEP) and catalyzing with 5-enolpyruvylshikimate-3-phosphate synthase enzyme. In the last reaction, 5-enolpyruvylshikimate-3-phosphate is converted to chorismate by the enzyme chorismate synthase [21, 23].

It forms anthranilate from chorismate formed in the last reaction of the shikimate pathway by giving amino group, which is part of the indole ring, in subsequent reactions for glutamine amino acid by way of the anthranilate synthase enzyme, which catalyzes the initial reaction of tryptophan biosynthesis [22]. N-(5′-phosphoribosyl) anthranilate is formed as a result of the elimination of pyrophosphate from phosphoribosyl-pyrophosphate (PRPP) by the enzyme anthranilate phosphoribosyltransferase. N-(5′-phosphoribosyl) anthranilate isomerase is responsible for the isomerization of N-(5′-phosphoribosyl) anthranilate to enol-1-o-carboxyphenylamino-1-deoxy-ribulose phosphate [24, 25].

Indole-3-glycerol-phosphate synthase catalyzes its conversion to indole-3-glycerol-phosphate by decarboxylating enol-1-o-carboxyphenylamino-1-deoxy-ribulose phosphate. In the last reaction, tryptophan synthase catalyzes the formation of tryptophan from indole-3-glycerol-phosphate by using indole and serine amino acids (**Figure 2**) [21, 26].

2.2 Synthesis of melatonin

Anabolism: Tryptophan is a nonpolar amino acid containing an indole ring [27]. Tryptophan amino acid, which is in the class of essential amino acids, is required to be taken from the diet through nutrition since it cannot be synthesized in humans and monogastric animals [20].

Melatonin, which is synthesized from the amino acid tryptophan, is synthesized in bacteria, unicellular eukaryotes, and plants. Melatonin is synthesized from retina, gastrointestinal system, kidney, liver, thyroid gland, bone marrow, leukocytes, membranous cochlea, placenta, Harderian gland, gonads, breast tissue, adrenal gland, lung, skin, adipose tissue, blood vessels, lymphocytes, neutrophils, lymphoid tissues, and some brain areas, is mainly synthesized from the pineal gland [28, 29].

The pineal gland plays an important role as a functional neuroendocrine transducer of photoperiodic changes that occur in environmental or seasonal events by activating N-acetyl transferase transfer [30]. Norepinephrine is the most important transmitter in the postganglionic sympathetic nerve endings in this gland. The suprachiasmatic nucleus (SCN), which is one of the nuclei that can receive signals from the retina through nerves during the day and in light, effectively inhibits the release of norepinephrine from these nerve endings [31, 32]. In the dark, the release

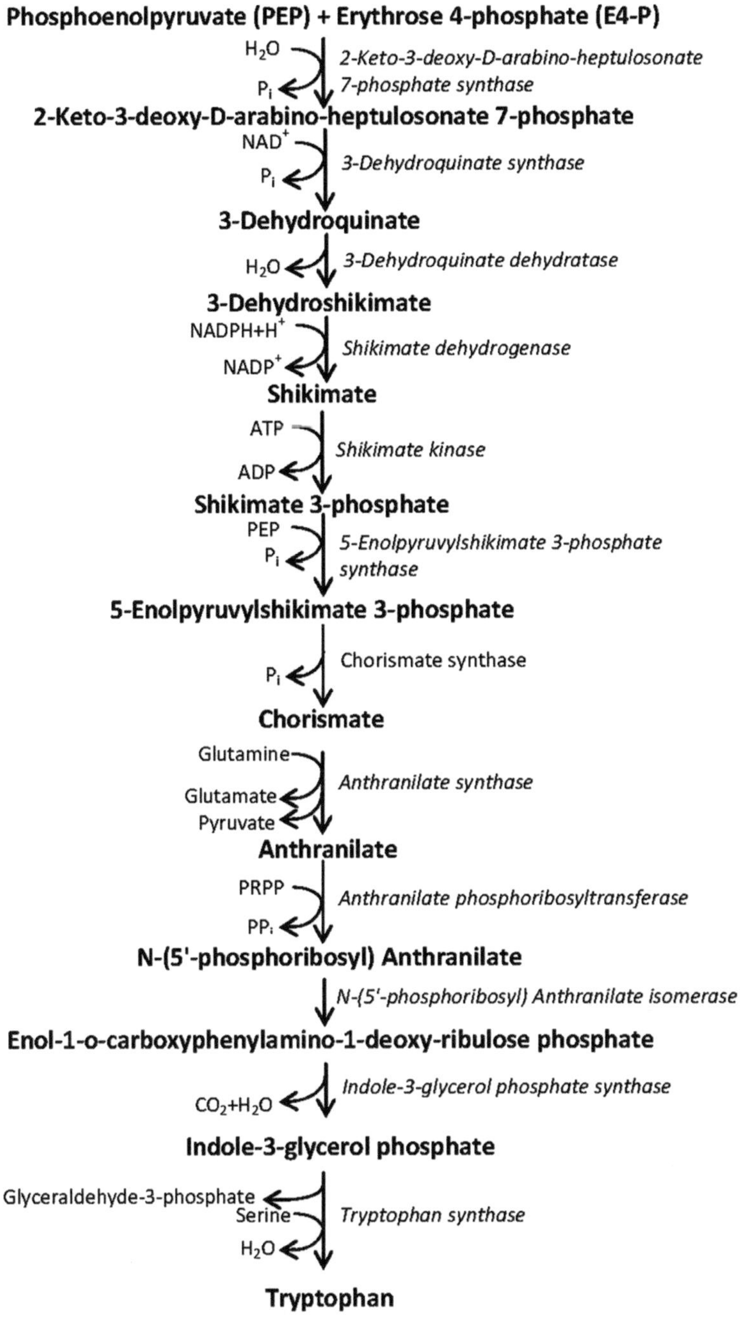

Figure 2.
Tryptophan synthesis.

of norepinephrine from the nerve endings begins. Norepinephrine then binds to β-adrenergic receptors on the pinealocyte membrane and causes an increase in intracellular cAMP. As a result, it increases the activity of the N-acetyltransferase enzyme, which is a rate-limiting enzyme in melatonin synthesis in increasing intracellular cAMP and melatonin synthesis increases from serotonin [30, 32].

Melatonin synthesis begins with the uptake of tryptophan from the circulatory system by pinealocytes [33]. While tryptophan is converted to 5-hydroxy-tryptophan by the tryptophan hydroxylase enzyme catalysis, 5-hydroxy-tryptophan is also converted to serotonin (5-hydroxy-tryptamine) via aromatic L-amino acid decarboxylase [34]. N-acetyl serotonin is formed with the catalysis of 5-hydroxy-tryptamine N-acetyltransferase enzyme. N-acetyl serotonin is converted into melatonin (N-acetyl-5-methoxy-tryptamine) by being methylated with the catalysis of 5-hydroxyindole-o-methyltransferase enzyme (**Figure 3**) [28, 35, 36].

Catabolism: Melatonin is metabolized by isoforms of cytochrome P450 mono-oxygenase enzymes (CYP1A2, CYP1A1, and CYP1B1) found in the liver. Of these isoforms, both CYP1A2 and CY2C19 enzymes can demethylate melatonin to N-acetyl serotonin or can convert melatonin to 6-hydroxymelatonin by hydroxylation [37]. The half-life of melatonin, of which 70% is transported to the liver depending on albumin, varies between 3 and 45 minutes [38]. Less than 1% of melatonin is reported to be excreted with urine as 6-sulphatoxymelatonin by conjugating lesser extent with glucuronic acid or mostly conjugating with sulfate for the rest (**Figure 3**) [39, 40].

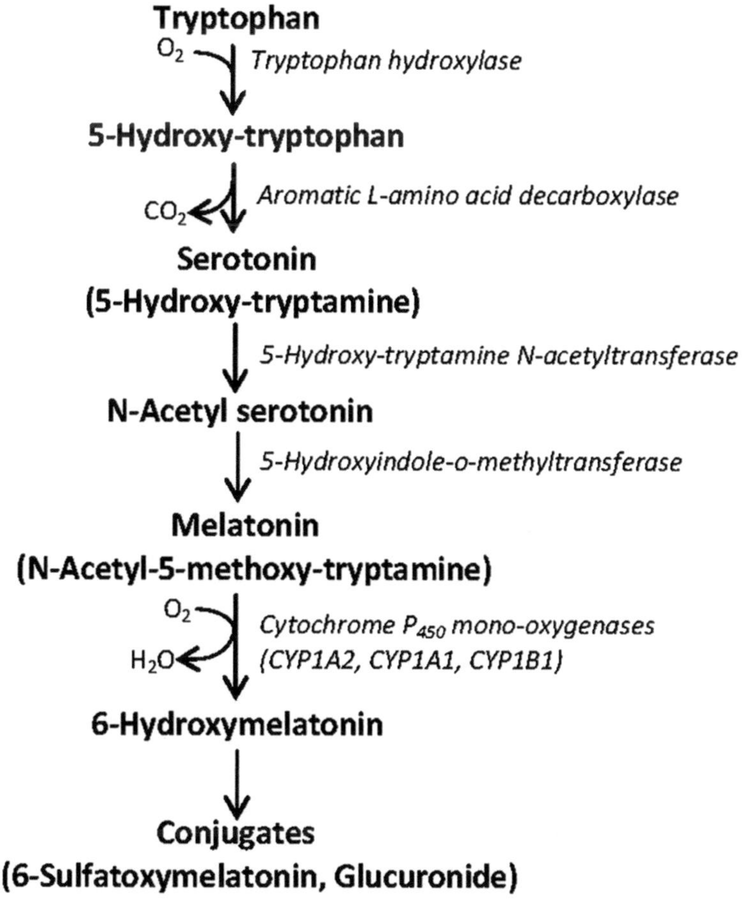

Figure 3.
Anabolism and catabolism of melatonin.

3. Antioxidant effects of melatonin

Free radicals, which are low molecular weight, short-lived and unstable structures, are highly active chemical structures that have unpaired electrons in their final orbits and try to share the electrons of other compounds to make up for this gap [41, 42]. Free radicals, which cause oxidation, are mainly oxygen-derived metabolites, superoxide anions (O_2^-), hydrogen peroxide (H_2O_2), hydroxyl radical (OH^-), and lipid peroxides [43]. Oxidative stress occurs as a result of increased reactive oxygen species (ROS) for various reasons and insufficient antioxidant mechanisms. Free radicals, which are formed by natural metabolic pathways in the body, are normally eliminated by radical scavenging antioxidant systems. Antioxidants are the molecules that prevent cell damage by inhibiting the formation of free radicals or scavenging existing radicals [44, 45]. While antioxidants can be classified according to their structure as those being enzymatic [superoxide dismutase (SOD), glutathione peroxidase (GPx), catalase (CAT), and glutathione-S-transferase (GST)] and non-enzymatic [Reduced glutathione (GSH), vitamin A, vitamin C, vitamin E, and melatonin], they can also be classified according to their cell localization as (i) intracellular antioxidants (SOD, CAT, and GPx), (ii) extracellular antioxidants (albumin, vitamin C, and urate) and (iii) membrane antioxidants (vitamin A and vitamin E) [46].

Melatonin hormone, which is a non-enzyme antioxidant, helps to eliminate harmful conditions stimulated by oxidative stress by inhibiting protein oxidation, lipid peroxidation, mitochondrial damage, and DNA degradation due to both its direct free radical scavenging activity and its contribution to the antioxidant defense system [47]. Melatonin, which is an antioxidant and was first suggested in 1991 by Ianaş et al., keeps radicals before the membrane and detoxifies them by protecting the membrane by attaching them to the outer surface of the cell membrane [48]. Melatonin hormone removes hydroxyl and oxygen radicals and inhibits nitric oxide synthase [49] and this feature of melatonin [50] that prevents lipid peroxidation reactions, especially by scavenging the $OH^{\cdot}$ radical, is due to the pyrrole ring in its structure [51]. Melatonin increases the levels of antioxidant enzymes, such as mitochondrial SOD, cytosolic SOD, GPx, and GSH in the cell [52]. In addition, it is a powerful antioxidant that prevents oxidative and nitrosative damage due to its ability to eliminate toxic oxygen derivatives formed in metabolic activities and reduces the formation of ROS and reactive nitrogen species [32, 53].

Melatonin shows its antioxidant effect in three ways. *(i) Direct antioxidant effect*: Blocking free radicals with the formation of N_1-Acetyl-N_2-formyl-5-methoxyquinuramine from the pyrrole ring of melatonin in the presence of free radicals [54–57], *(ii) Indirect antioxidant effect*: Suppressing oxidative stress by increasing the activity of enzymes, such as SOD, GPx, and GSH [54, 55], and *(iii) Effect via prooxidant enzyme*: Reducing free radical formation as a result of suppressing some prooxidant enzymes [48].

Antioxidant properties of melatonin have been shown in the studies conducted [58–62]. It has been reported that melatonin is at least two times more effective antioxidant than vitamin E and five times more effective than glutathione [55]. In the studies conducted, it is known that when melatonin is applied together with vitamin E and vitamin C, better protection is obtained than when applied alone [63] and melatonin has a suppressive effect on the formation of free radicals formed during electron transport in mitochondria. Melatonin reduces the formation of destructive toxic hydroxyl radicals by chelating transition metals taking place in Fenton/Haber-Weiss reactions [64]. It protects the biomolecules found in the whole structure of the cell against free radical formation by reacting with toxic hydroxyl radicals. Melatonin forms a non-enzymatic defense mechanism against the destructive properties of hydroxyl radicals and is more effective than other known antioxidants in protecting the organism against oxidative damage. It terminates lipid peroxidation by capturing the peroxide radical unlike antioxidants, such as ascorbic acid, alpha-tocopherol, and GSH. It has been reported that liver, kidney, and brain tissue glutathione peroxidase activity in rats increased after the administration of melatonin. Significant decreases in liver, lung, brain tissue, and glutathione peroxidase activity were reported in rats for which pinealectomy is made [48].

Many studies examining the effects on the synthesis and circulating amount of nitric oxide (NO), which is an important molecule of melatonin that plays a role in many physiological and physiopathological events, have been done. The physiological effect of NO occurs when soluble guanylate cyclase is activated to form cGMP. Decreased melatonin level causes decreased guanylate cyclase activity in many tissues. As a result, the cGMP level decreases, and the cAMP level increases. Thus, cell membrane thickness and rigidity increase, and degenerative damage formation accelerates [65]. When the relationship between NO and melatonin is examined, it has been suggested that the peroxynitrite anion, which is formed as a result of the reaction between NO and nitrosomelatonin and the reaction of NO and O_2 in the presence of O_2, is also occupied by melatonin [66, 67].

Unlike other antioxidants, it does not have a toxic effect in excessive use. Melatonin differs from classical antioxidants in various aspects and turns into less harmful pro-oxidant substances from the oxidants whose effects they abolish. However, after melatonin effects oxidant substances, is also effective as antioxidants in the intermediate stages and the resulting products. This property is very valuable as an antioxidant agent and is characterized as a "suicidal or terminal antioxidant" [68]. Melatonin reduces the synthesis of adhesion molecules and proinflammatory cytokines [69, 70]. Melatonin prevents linoleic acid, which is an energy source and growth factor of melatonin, which promotes the repair of damaged DNA, from entering the cell and suppresses its metabolism [71, 72].

4. Conclusion

The shikimate pathway, used by bacteria, fungi, algae, and plants, is a seven-step metabolic pathway for the biosynthesis of aromatic amino acids. However, this pathway is absent in animals. For this reason, melatonin, a neurohormone synthesized from tryptophan, an essential amino acid that must be taken with food, is synthesized by the retina, bone marrow, and gastrointestinal system, mainly by the pineal gland. Melatonin plays a role in the regulation of many physiological and biological functions in animals, such as the regulation of sleep time, blood pressure, and breeding season. In addition, due to its small molecular size and high lipophilic, it can reach all organelles of the cell and cross the blood–brain barrier. In addition, melatonin, which is a powerful antioxidant, provides direct scavenging of hydroxyl and oxygen radicals with high toxicity and stimulates antioxidant enzymes.

Author details

Oguz Merhan
Faculty of Veterinary, Department of Biochemistry, Kafkas University, Kars, Turkey

*Address all correspondence to: oguzmerhan@hotmail.com

References

[1] Molaakbari E, Mostafavi A, Beitollahi H. Simultaneous electrochemical determination of dopamine, melatonin, methionine and caffeine. Sensors and Actuators B: Chemical. 2015;**208**:195-203. DOI: 10.1016/j.snb.2014.10.130

[2] Sun R, Wang Y, He H, Wan Y, Li L, Sha J, et al. Solubility measurement, solubility behavior analysis and thermodynamic modelling of melatonin in twelve pure solvents from 278.15 K to 323.15 K. Journal of Molecular Liquids. 2020;**319**:114139

[3] Babaei A, Taheri AR, Farahani IK. Nanomolar simultaneous determination of levodopa and melatonin at a new cobalt hydroxide nanoparticles and multi-walled carbon nanotubes composite modified carbon ionic liquid electrode. Sensors and Actuators B. 2013;**183**:265-272. DOI: 10.1016/j.snb.2013.03.101

[4] Beyer CE, Steketee JD, Saphier D. Antioxidant properties of melatonin-an emerging mystery. Biochemical Pharmacology. 1998;**56**:1265-1272. DOI: 10.1016/s0006-2952(98)00180-4

[5] Zawilska JB, Skene DJ, Arendt J. Physiology and pharmacology of melatonin in relation to biological rhythms. Pharmacological Reports. 2009;**61**:383-410. DOI: 10.1016/s1734-1140(09)70081-7

[6] Pevet P. Melatonin. Dialogues in Clinical Neuroscience. 2002;**4**:57-72. DOI: 10.31887/DCNS.2002.4.1/ppevet

[7] Grivas TB, Savvidou OD. Melatonin the "light of night" in human biology and adolescent idiopathic scoliosis. Scoliosis. 2007;**2**:6. DOI: 10.1186/1748-7161-2-6

[8] Wood S, Loudon A. Clocks for all seasons: Unwinding the roles and mechanisms of circadian and interval timers in the hypothalamus and pituitary. The Journal of Endocrinology. 2014;**222**:R39-R59. DOI: 10.1530/JOE-14-0141

[9] Claustrat B, Leston J. Melatonin: Physiological effects in humans. Neuro-Chirurgie. 2015;**61**:77-84. DOI: 10.1016/j.neuchi.2015.03.002

[10] Hower IM, Harper SA, Buford TW. Circadian rhythms, exercise, and cardiovascular health. Journal of Circadian Rhythms. 2018;**16**:1-8. DOI: 10.5334/jcr.164

[11] Chan S, Debono M. Replication of cortisol circadian rhythm: New advances in hydrocortisone replacement therapy. Therapeutic Advances in Endocrinology and Metabolism. 2010;**1**:129-138. DOI: 10.1177/2042018810380214

[12] Fatima G, Sharma VP, Verma NS. Circadian variations in melatonin and cortisol in patients with cervical spinal cord injury. Spinal Cord. 2016;**54**:364-367. DOI: 10.1038/sc.2015.176

[13] Cevik C, Aslan R. Effects of photoperiod variations and alpha-lipoic acid treatment on melatonin, cortisol, and oxidative stress levels in the blood of rats. Turkish Journal of Biology. 2015;**39**:941-949. DOI: 10.3906/biy-1506-77

[14] O'Callaghan D. A practical approach to the management of reproductive seasonality in sheep. Reproduction in Domestic Animals. 1999;**34**:285-291

[15] Carcangiu V, Mura MC, Parmeggiani A, Piccione G, Bini PP,

Cosso G, et al. Daily rhythm of blood melatonin concentrations in sheep of different ages. Biological Rhythm Research. 2013;**44**:908-915. DOI: 10.1080/09291016.2013.781317

[16] Molik E, Błasiak M, Misztal T, Romanowicz K, Zieba DA. Profile of gonadotropic hormone secretion in sheep with disturbed rhythm of seasonality. Czech Journal of Animal Science. 2017;**62**:242-248. DOI: 10.17221/22/2016-CJAS

[17] deNicolo G, Morris ST, Kenyon PR, Morel PCH, Parkinson TJ. Melatonin-improved reproductive performance in sheep bred out of season. Animal Reproduction Science. 2008;**109**:124-133. DOI: 10.1016/j.anireprosci.2007.10.012

[18] Rosa HJD, Bryant MJ. Seasonality of reproduction in sheep. Small Ruminant Research. 2003;**48**:155-171. DOI: 10.1016/S0921-4488(03)00038-5

[19] Uyar A, Alan M. The effect of melatonin applied in early anestrous season on ovulation and pregnancy rates in ewes. The Journal of The Faculty of Veterinary Medicine University of Yuzuncu Yil. 2008;**19**:47-54

[20] Tzin V, Galili G. The biosynthetic pathways for shikimate and aromatic amino acids in *Arabidopsis thaliana*. The Arabidopsis Book. 2010;**8**:e0132. DOI: 10.1199/tab. 0132

[21] Maeda H, Dudareva N. The shikimate pathway and aromatic amino acid biosynthesis in plants. Annual Review of Plant Biology. 2012;**63**:73-105. DOI: 10.1146/annurev-arplant-042811-105439

[22] Parthasarathy A, Cross PJ, Dobson RCJ, Adams LE, Savka MA, Hudson AO. A three-ring circus: Metabolism of the three proteogenic aromatic amino acids and their role in the health of plants and animals. Frontiers in Molecular Biosciences. 2018;**5**:29. DOI: 10.3389/fmolb.2018.00029

[23] Yokoyama R, de Oliveira MVV, Kleven B, Maeda HA. The entry reaction of the plant shikimate pathway is subjected to highly complex metabolite-mediated regulation. The Plant Cell. 2021;**33**:671-696. DOI: 10.1093/plcell/koaa042

[24] Radwanski ER, Last RL. Tryptophan biosynthesis and metabolism: Biochemical and molecular genetics. The Plant Cell. 1995;**7**:921-934. DOI: 10.1105/tpc.7.7.921

[25] Sinha SC, Smith JL. The PRT protein family. Current Opinion in Structural Biology. 2001;**11**:733-739. DOI: 10.1016/S0959-440X(01)00274-3

[26] Yanofsky C. RNA-based regulation of genes of tryptophan synthesis and degradation, in bacteria. RNA. 2007;**13**:1141-1154. DOI: 10.1261/rna.620507

[27] Barik S. The uniqueness of tryptophan in biology: Properties, metabolism, interactions and localization in proteins. International Journal of Molecular Sciences. 2020;**21**:8776. DOI: 10.3390/ijms21228776

[28] Srinivasan V, Spence DW, Pandi Perumal SR, Trakht I, Esquifino AI, Cardinali DP, et al. Melatonin, environmental light, and breast cancer. Breast Cancer Research and Treatment. 2008;**108**:339-350. DOI: 10.1007/s10549-007-9617-5

[29] Hardeland R, Cardinali DP, Srinivasan V, Spence DW, Brown GM, PandiPerumalSR.Melatonin-apleiotropic, orchestrating regulator molecule. Progress in Neurobiology.

2011;**93**:350-384. DOI: 10.1016/j.pneurobio.2010.12.004

[30] Pampori ZA, Sheikh AA, Aarif O, Hasin D, Bhat IA. Physiology of reproductive seasonality in sheep – an update. Biological Rhythm Research. 2018;**586-598**. DOI: 10.1080/09291016.2018.1548112

[31] Schomerus C, Korf HW. Mechanisms regulating melatonin synthesis in the mammalian pineal organ. Annals of the New York Academy of Sciences. 2005;**1057**:372-383. DOI: 10.1196/annals.1356.028

[32] Singh M, Jadhav HR. Melatonin: Functions and ligands. Drug Discovery Today. 2014;**19**:1410-1418. DOI: 10.1016/j.drudis.2014.04.014

[33] Cagnacci A. Melatonin in relation to physiology in adult humans. Journal of Pineal Research. 1996;**21**:200-213

[34] Erdag D, Merhan O, Yildiz B. Biochemical and pharmacological properties of biogenic amines. In: Proestos C, editor. Biogenic Amines. London: InTechOpen; 2019. pp. 63-76. DOI: 10.5772/intechopen.81569

[35] Tan DX, Manchester LC, Sanchez-Barcelo E, Mediavilla MD, Reiter RJ. Significance of high levels of endogenous melatonin in mammalian cerebrospinal fluid and in the central nervous system. Current Neuropharmacology. 2010;**8**:162-167. DOI: 10.2174/157015910792246182

[36] Zhao D, Yu Y, Shen Y, Liu Q, Zhao Z, Sharma R, et al. Melatonin synthesis and function: Evolutionary history in animals and plants. Frontiers in Endocrinology. 2019;**10**:249. DOI: 10.3389/fendo.2019.00249

[37] Pandi Perumal SR, Srinivasan V, Maestroni GJM, Cardinali DP, Poeggeler B, Hardeland R. Melatonin: Nature's most versatile biological signal. The FEBS Journal. 2006;**273**:2813-2838. DOI: 10.1111/j.1742-4658.2006.05322.x

[38] Macchi MM, Bruce JN. Human pineal physiology and functional significance of melatonin. Frontiers in Neuroendocrinology. 2004;**25**:177-195. DOI: 10.1016/j.yfrne.2004.08.001

[39] Paakkonen T, Makinen TM, Leppaluoto J, Vakkuri O, Rintamaki H, Palinkas LA, et al. Urinary melatonin: A noninvasive method to follow human pineal function as studied in three experimental conditions. Journal of Pineal Research. 2006;**40**:110-115. DOI: 10.1111/j.1600-079X.2005.00300.x

[40] Hardeland R. Melatonin metabolism in the central nervous system. Current Neuropharmacology. 2010;**8**:168-181. DOI: 10.2174/157015910792246244

[41] Halliwell B. The wanderings of a free radical. Free Radical Biology and Medicine. 2009;**46**:531-542. DOI: 10.1016/j.freeradbiomed.2008.11.008

[42] Lobo V, Patil A, Phatak A, Chandra N. Free radicals, antioxidants and functional foods: İmpact on human health. Pharmacognosy Reviews. 2010;**4**:118-126. DOI: 10.4103/0973-7847.70902

[43] Kohen R, Nyska A. Oxidation of biological systems: Oxidative stress phenomena, antioxidants, redox reactions, and methods for their quantification. Toxicologic Pathology. 2002;**30**:620-650. DOI: 10.1080/01926230290166724

[44] Kahkönen MP, Hopia AI, Vuorela HJ, Rauha JP, Pihlaja K, Kujala TS, et al. Antioxidant activity of plant extracts containing phenolic compounds. Journal of Agricultural and Food Chemistry.

1999;**47**:3954-3962. DOI: 10.1021/jf990146l

[45] Touitou Y. Human aging and melatonin. Clinical relevance. Experimental Gerontology. 2001;**36**:1083-1100. DOI: 10.1016/s0531-5565(01)00120-6

[46] Gutteridge JM. Lipid peroxidation and antioxidants as biomarkers of tissue damage. Clinical Chemistry. 1995;**41**:1819-1828

[47] Galano A, Castaneda-Arriaga R, Perez-Gonzalez A, Tan DX, Reiter RJ. Phenolic melatonin-related compounds: Their role as chemical protectors against oxidative stress. Molecules. 2016;**21**:1442. DOI: 10.3390/molecules21111442

[48] Reiter R, Tang L, Garcia JJ, Munoz-Hoyos A. Pharmacological actions of melatonin in oxygen radical pathophysiology. Life Sciences. 1997;**60**:2255-2271. DOI: 10.1016/s0024-3205(97)00030-1

[49] Ravindra T, Lakshmi NK, Ahuja YR. Melatonin in pathogenesis and therapy of cancer. Indian Journal of Medical Sciences. 2006;**60**:523-535

[50] Abuja PM, Albertini R. Methods for monitoring oxidative stress, lipid peroxidation and oxidation resistance of lipoproteins. Clinica Chimica Acta. 2001;**306**:1-17. DOI: 10.1016/s0009-8981(01)00393-x

[51] Atasoy N. Melatonin and antioxidant effects. Journal of Duzce University Health Sciences Institute. 2019;**9**:196-201. DOI: 10.33631/duzcesbed.492547

[52] Huang CC, Lai CJ, Tsai MH, Wu YC, Chen KT, Jou MJ, et al. Effects of melatonin on the nitric oxide system and protein nitration in the hypobaric hypoxic rat hippocampus. BMC Neuroscience. 2015;**16**:61. DOI: 10.1186/s12868-015-0199-6

[53] Pevet P, Klosen P, Felder-Schmittbuhl MP. The hormone melatonin: Animal studies. Best Practice and Research. Clinical Endocrinology and Metabolism. 2017;**31**:547-559. DOI: 10.1016/j.beem.2017.10.010

[54] Reiter RJ, Tan DX, Osuna C, Gitto E. Actions of melatonin in the reduction of oxidative stress. A review. Journal of Biomedical Science. 2000;**7**:444-458. DOI: 10.1007/BF02253360

[55] Reiter RJ, Tan DX, Mayo JC, Sainz RM, Leon J, Czarnocki Z. Melatonin as an antioxidant: Biochemical mechanisms and pathophysiological implications in humans. Acta Biochimica Polonica. 2003;**50**:1129-1146

[56] Tomas Zapico C, Coto MA. Melatonin as antioxidant under pathological processes. Recent Patents on Endocrine, Metabolic and Immune Drug Discovery. 2007;**1**:63-82. DOI: 10.2174/187221407779814561

[57] Chrustek A, Olszewska SD. Melatonin as a powerful antioxidant. Acta Pharmaceutica - Sciendo. 2021;**71**:335-354. DOI: 10.2478/acph-2021-0027

[58] Poeggeler B, Saarela S, Reiter RJ, Tan DX, Chen LD, Manchester LC, et al. Melatonin-a highly potent endogenous radical scavenger and electron donor: New aspects of the oxidation chemistry of this indole accessed *in vitro*. Annals of the New York Academy of Sciences. 1994;**738**:419-4120. DOI: 10.1111/j.1749-6632.1994.tb21831.x

[59] Marshall KA, Reiter RJ, Poeggeler B, Aruoma OI, Halliwell B. Evaluation of the antioxidant activity of melatonin *in vitro*. Free Radical Biology and Medicine.

1996;**21**:307-315. DOI: 10.1016/0891-5849(96)00046-9

[60] Arnao MB, Hernandez RJ. The physiological function of melatonin in plants. Plant Signaling and Behavior. 2006;**1**:89-95. DOI: 10.4161/psb.1.3.2640

[61] Kara A, Akman S, Ozkanlar S, Tozoglu U, Kalkan Y, Canakci CF, et al. Immune modulatory and antioxidant effects of melatonin in experimental periodontitis in rats. Free Radical Biology and Medicine. 2013;**55**:21-26. DOI: 10.1016/j.freeradbiomed.2012.11.002

[62] Emamgholipour S, Hossein-Nezhad A, Sahraian MA, Askarisadr F, Ansari M. Evidence for possible role of melatonin in reducing oxidative stress in multiple sclerosis through its effect on SIRT1 and antioxidant enzymes. Life Sciences. 2016;**145**:34-41. DOI: 10.1016/j.lfs.2015.12.014

[63] Rohr UD, Herold J. Melatonin deficiencies in women. Maturitas. 2002;**1**:S85-S104. DOI: 10.1016/s0378-5122(02)00017-8

[64] Reiter RJ, Mayo JC, Tan DX, Sainz RM, Alatorre Jimenez M, Qin L. Melatonin as an antioxidant: Under promises but over delivers. Journal of Pineal Research. 2016;**61**:253-278. DOI: 10.1111/jpi.12360

[65] Peschke E, Bahr I, Mühlbauer E. Experimental and clinical aspects of melatonin and clock genes in diabetes. Journal of Pineal Research. 2015;**59**:1-23. DOI: 10.1111/jpi.12240

[66] Aydogan S, Yerer MB, Goktas A. Melatonin and nitric oxide. Journal of Endocrinological Investigation. 2006;**29**:281-287. DOI: 10.1007/BF03345555

[67] Hardeland R. Melatonin, its metabolites and their interference with reactive nitrogen compounds. Molecules. 2021;**26**:4105. DOI: 10.3390/molecules26134105

[68] Tan DX, Manchester LC, Reiter RJ, Qi WB, Karbownik M, Calvo JR. Significance of melatonin in antioxidative defense system: Reactions and products. Biological Signals and Receptors. 2000;**9**:137-159. DOI: 10.1159/000014635

[69] Reiter RJ. Melatonin: Clinical relevance. Best Practice and Research. Clinical Endocrinology and Metabolism. 2003;**17**:273-285. DOI: 10.1016/s1521-690x(03)00016-2

[70] Bantounou M, Plascevic J, Galley HF. Melatonin and related compounds: Antioxidant and anti-inflammatory actions. Antioxidants (Basel). 2022;**11**:532. DOI: 10.3390/antiox11030532

[71] Hill SM, Belancio VP, Dauchy RT, Xiang S, Brimer S, Mao L, et al. Melatonin: An inhibitor of breast cancer. Endocrine Related Cancer. 2015;**22**:R183-R204. DOI: 10.1530/ERC-15-0030

[72] Kohandel Z, Farkhondeh T, Aschner M, Samarghandian S. Molecular targets for the management of gastrointestinal cancer using melatonin, a natural endogenous body hormone. Biomedicine and Pharmacotherapy. 2021;**140**:111782. DOI: 10.1016/j.biopha.2021.111782

Section 4

The Role of Melatonin in Various Diseases

Chapter 4

A Promising Challenge in the Link between Melatonin and Breast Cancer: Exploring the Microbiome-Gut-Brain Axis

Alicia González-González, Aurora Laborda-Illanes, Soukaina Boutriq, Lidia Sánchez-Alcoholado, Daniel Castellano-Castillo, Isaac Plaza-Andrades, Jesús Peralta-Linero and María Isabel Queipo-Ortuño

Abstract

In this chapter, we describe the possible link between gut microbiota, melatonin, and breast cancer disease. It is widely described that changes in melatonin production due to circadian disruption is one of the causes of breast cancer. In addition, recently it is described that dysbiosis caused by changes in the gut microbiota composition could be as well constitute an important factor to induce breast cancer. The dysbiosis process, in turn, induces the stimulation of kynurenine pathway, leading to reduced circulating melatonin levels. Therefore, in this chapter we deep into the relationship between circadian disruption, dysbiosis, and breast cancer disease. This constitutes an important step in the therapeutic approach and prevention of this pathology.

Keywords: melatonin, breast cancer, gut microbiota, circadian disruption, dysbiosis, estrogens, estrobolome, anticancer therapies

1. Introduction

Breast cancer is one of the most common neoplasia in women, representing about 25% of all most cancer instances in women, and is the second main purpose of most cancer deaths in advanced countries [1]. The search for therapies for this pathology is an expanding field in medical research.

Melatonin is an indoleamine secreted in particular with the aid of using the pineal gland with circadian rhythmicity. Melatonin represents one of the links between circadian disruption and cancer development. The role of this hormone in the regulation of cancer cell growth has been extensively investigated and many studies have pointed out the oncostatic properties of melatonin against different neoplasia, including breast cancer, ovarian, skin, lymphomas, leukemia, sarcoma, hepatocarcinoma, colorectal cancer, melanoma, lung cancer, endometrial and cervical cancer, prostate cancer, larynx carcinoma, neural tumors, and pancreatic cancer [2]. Melatonin production takes place mainly during the night in the pineal gland. However, its synthesis is also produced in other parts of the body, including gastrointestinal tract [3]. Specifically, gut cells synthesize great quantities of this indoleamine [4]. Apart from this, melatonin can be produced by gut microbiota directly or indirectly, since microbiota produces short-chain fatty acids (SCFAs), which stimulate serotonin production. Serotonin by the action of two enzymes (arylalkylamine-N-acetyltransferase (AANAT) together with 14–3-3 proteins for its stabilization, and acetylserotonin O-methyltransferase (ASMT)) is converted into melatonin [5].

The melatonergic pathway starts with the uptake of tryptophan (Trp) [6]. This important amino acid is needed for lifestyle and growth, however, is not synthesized via way of means of the organism. In the body, Trp is transported around the periphery either bounded to albumin (90%) or in free form (10%) [7]. Trp can act as a precursor of different pathways once in the central nervous system (CNS). First, kynurenine pathway constitutes the major catabolism route (95% of whole Trp dietary intake) [8]. In second place, 3% of Trp is converted into tryptamine by decarboxylation or into indol-3-pyruvic acid by transamination. Thirdly, about 1% of Trp is used for protein synthesis, and finally, the melatonergic pathway is over 1% of whole Trp intake, being this route through which serotonin and melatonin synthesis is done [9].

The kynurenine pathway begins with the action of the rate-limiting enzymes Trp-2,3-dioxygenase (TDO) and indoleamine-2,3-dioxygenase (IDO-1 and IDO-2) [10]. TDO is an enzyme that is mainly expressed in the liver, apart from other organs such as the brain, where it is found in low quantities. TDO expression is induced by oxidative stress [9, 10]. In contrast, IDO-1 is found primarily in extrahepatic tissues such as the lungs, brain, or kidneys [9, 10]. IDO-1 expression is induced by lipopolysaccharides (LPS), amyloid peptides, human immunodeficiency virus (HIV) proteins [10], tumor necrosis factor-alpha (TNF-α), interferon gamma (IFN-γ), and by different proinflammatory cytokines, including interleukin-1beta (IL-1 β), IL-6, and IL-18 [8]. Thanks to the action of TDO and IDO, Trp is converted into kynurenine (KYN), which activates the aryl hydrocarbon receptor (AhR) [9]. After this activation, AhR/cytochrome P450 (CYP1B1) pathway starts, being this pathway fundamental in breast cancer [11]. After, CYP1B1 stimulates N-acetylserotonin (NAS) conversion from melatonin, causing an increase in NAS/melatonin ratio and a reduction in melatonin levels [12]. NAS induces the dimerization and activation of tyrosine kinase B receptors (TrkB) and the stimulation of the AKT and extracellular signal-regulated protein kinases 1 and 2 (ERK1/2) pathways [13], which are implicated in the survival, proliferation, invasion, and migration of breast cancer cells and their resistance to the different therapies.

As previously described, the kynurenine pathway is implicated in the development of breast cancer. Apart from this, it has been implicated in a wide range of diseases and disorders, including inflammatory processes, infectious diseases, neurological disorders, Huntington's disease, affective disorders, autoimmune diseases, peripheral conditions, and cancer progression. A key indicator of cancer progression is often the upregulation in IDO-1, resulting in an accelerated and sustained degradation in Trp [8]. Tryptophan degradation products through the kynurenine pathway exhibit neuromodulatory and inflammatory effects and have been related to cancer development and tumor progression [9]. Glioblastoma sufferers with a high-ratio KYN/Trp had a bad evolution and occasional survival as compared with sufferers with a decrease ratio [14].

The importance of the kynurenine pathway during cancer development has encouraged recent studies on the use of IDO inhibitors as a therapeutic strategy for treatment of breast, lung, and ovarian cancer [9]. Suppression of IDO and TDO would lead to a decrease in kynurenine production [15]. It is a novel therapeutic target in cancer research and the results have been positive. Using transgenic mouse model of breast cancer, IDO-1 inhibitors, 1-methyltryptophan (1-MT), and methyl-thiohydantoin-tryptophan were able to potentiate the efficacy of chemotherapy drugs, promoting tumor regression without increasing the side effects [16]. 1-MT, a competitive IDO inhibitor, has been tested and approved in phase I clinical trials in patients with metastatic neoplasms as well as in lung, ovarian, Fallopian tube, and breast cancers displaying sickness stabilization in many cases [17–20].

In addition, the alterations in the melatonergic pathway that occurred in breast cancer cells produce changes in gut permeability and microbiome composition accompanied by a reduction in butyrate levels and an increase in LPS, leading to a pro-inflammatory response, and increasing the production of Trp catabolites, thus decreasing the melatonin production [21].

Therefore, a bidirectional flow is observed between alterations in the composition of the microbiota (dysbiosis), the production of melatonin levels (circadian disruption), and breast cancer. Thus, in this chapter, we will deal with the properties of melatonin, highlighting its antiestrogenic properties, and its relationship with the microbiota and breast cancer.

2. Melatonin interaction molecules

Melatonin has different actions depending on its binding to specific receptors. On the one hand, melatonin activates MT1, MT2, and MT3 cell membrane receptors coupled to Gi protein [22]. This hormone binds to these receptors, reducing cAMP levels, thus counteracting the estrogen-induced estrogen receptor alpha (ERα) transcriptional activity by interacting with the cAMP signaling cascade [22] and thus suppressing adenylate cyclase [23].

On the other hand, melatonin binds to calmodulin (CaM), behaving as an antagonist capable of binding and inactivating the Ca2+/CaM complex. CaM is important in the activation of ERα, by facilitating its association with other coactivators and binding to the estrogen response element (ERE) [24]. Melatonin inactivates the Ca2+/CaM complex, inhibiting CAM-dependent estradiol-induced transactivation of the ER [25].

Besides, melatonin interacts with the retinoic Z receptor/retinoid, receptor-related orphan nuclear receptor alpha and beta (RZR/RORα and RORβ) superfamily. The estrogen-induced transcriptional activity of ERα is due to the overexpression of these receptors and its effects can be inhibited by melatonin by the activation of MT1 or by inhibiting CaM [26].

Finally, melatonin is described as an antioxidant. It transfers electrons to hydroxyl radicals, superoxide anions, hydrogen peroxide, hypochlorous acid, nitric oxide, and peroxynitric anions [27]. Furthermore, melatonin stimulates the expression of antioxidant enzymes, being a powerful free radical scavenger [28, 29].

2.1 Melatonin actions in cancer

Melatonin has been widely described in the literature as a potential antitumor agent due to its several antitumoral properties [30]. Firstly, melatonin is a powerful antioxidant molecule that neutralizes the free radicals that induce carcinogen modifications in the DNA and cause cell nuclear damage, preventing the appearance of cancer [31].

Secondly, melatonin is known to prevent circadian disruption that occurs frequently in women who work night shifts by exposure to artificial light at night (ALAN) [32]. Therefore, this hormone synchronizes the circadian rhythms with ambient light [33].

Furthermore, melatonin regulates fat metabolism since it prevents the linoleic acid adsorption. This fatty acid activates the epidermal growth factor (EGF), mitogen-activated kinases (MAPK), and ERK1/2 pathways, promoting the proliferation and growth of the tumor. Thus, melatonin can prevent cancer by inhibiting the acid linoleic adsorption [30].

On the other hand, melatonin is known to regulate cell cycle. The Trp-derivated causes the arrest of cell cycle by lengthening the GAP1 (G1) growth phase, thus delaying the entrance to the synthesis (S) and mitosis (M) phases [34]. For this reason, melatonin has antiproliferative actions. Besides, melatonin stimulates apoptosis process of the tumoral cells by increasing p53 expression [35, 36].

Also, low levels of melatonin are related to alterations in the immune system [33]. Melatonin stimulates immune system mediated by interleukins and other cytokines in monocytes and lymphocytes, reducing tumor cell survival and proliferation [28].

Apart from these antitumoral actions, melatonin inhibits angiogenesis by avoiding the different steps in this process. In fact, this hormone inhibits invasion, migration [37], and metastasis of tumoral cells [38], thus preventing tumoral cells from entering to the vascular system and inhibiting tumoral angiogenesis [39].

Additionally, melatonin also inhibits telomerase activity, which is stimulated in breast cancer cells [40]. Telomerase activity is responsible to maintain the DNA stability, contributing to the cancer cells' immortality, and providing an unlimited capacity for the division of neoplastic cells [30]. Melatonin prevents the action of estrogen, cadmium, or estradiol-induced telomerase reverse transcriptase (hTERT) transcription in the breast cancer cells and reduces the transactivation of hTERT initiated by ERα [41].

Finally, melatonin is known to be a potent antiestrogenic molecule by acting on the neuroendocrine-reproductive axis and preventing the estrogen actions that at last will cause breast cancer [30]. In the next section, we will deal with the actions of melatonin behaving as a selective estrogen modulator (SERM) or selective estrogen enzyme modulator (SEEM) in detail.

2.2 Melatonin as a natural antiestrogen molecule

Melatonin is a molecule that modifies the estrogen levels by altering the estrogen synthesis pathway preventing breast cancer. This hormone has direct actions at the level of the tumoral cell, behaving as a SERM [42]. On the one hand, it counteracts the effects of estrogen acting as a natural antiestrogen. Besides, melatonin binds to the MT1 receptor and avoids the binding between the estradiol (E2)-ERα complex to ERE and the initiation of transcription [25]. In addition, the literature has described another mechanism by which melatonin binds to calmodulin (CaM), preventing the binding of the E2-ERα complex to ERE and thus its transcription [25].

On the other hand, melatonin modulates the expression and activity of the different enzymes implies in the synthesis of estrogens (SEEM), thus reducing its levels. In concrete, melatonin reduces the expression and activity of aromatase, sulfatase

(STS), and 17β-hydroxysteroid dehydrogenase (17βHSD) enzymes and enhances the expression and activity of estrogen sulfotransferase (EST). Aromatase is the enzyme responsible to convert the androgens into estrogens by the stimulation of its different promoters (promoter II, I.3 and I.4) [43]. Melatonin is able to inhibit this enzyme by inhibiting cyclooxygenase-2 (COX-2) and decreasing the production of prostaglandin E2 (PGE2), which reduces the levels of cAMP and indirectly decreases the activation of aromatase promoters and finally decreases the aromatase expression and activity, which will reduce the estrogen levels [44]. 17βHSD and sulfatase enzymes are the responsible for the conversion of biologically inactive estrogens into their active form. EST is the enzyme responsible to do the opposite action, converting the steroids into the active form [45]. Therefore, melatonin by modulating the expression and activity of these enzymes can prevent the development of breast cancer by reducing theestrogen levels [43].

Finally, melatonin has indirect actions on the hypothalamus-hypophysis-gonads axis, lowering the synthesis of ovarian estrogens and prolactin, which are fundamental in mammary growth [28].

3. Melatonin and breast cancer

Cohen et al. proposed that a reduction in melatonin levels induced an increase in estrogen levels, being the cause of the development of breast cancer [46]. Since then, there are numerous research that display the association between melatonin levels, estrogens and cancer progression [39]. There are studies in which women with low levels of circulating melatonin, suffer from breast cancer [28]. Specially, women with tumors with positive receptors to estrogen or progesterone, have lower nocturnal levels of melatonin than those with negative hormone receptors [47]. Furthermore, lower levels of 6-sulfatexymelatonin in the urine of breast cancer patients are observed, in comparison with women with benign pathologies [48]. Apart from this, it is described that shift work produces circadian disruption, reducing the production of melatonin and thus increasing the risk of breast cancer [30].

The uses of melatonin are demonstrated *in vitro*, *in vivo* and in some clinical trials. In regard to the *in vitro* studies, melatonin inhibits the proliferation of MCF-7 breast cancer cells through the inhibition of ERα [30]. Regarding the *in vivo* studies, most of them were performed in mice with mammary adenocarcinomas induced by chemical carcinogens [49]. In these studies, mice treated with melatonin, showed inhibition of mammary tumor growth [50]. Finally, most of the clinical trials with melatonin in cancer patients have been made by Lissoni and colleagues [51]. They demonstrated that melatonin can extend survival in metastatic cancer patients [51].

3.1 Fat tissue, estrogens and breast cancer

The link between obesity and breast cancer has been widely described in the literature. Obesity consists of excessive fat accumulation in white adipose tissue (WAT) in addition to hyperplasia and hypertrophy of adipocytes. These events cause chronic inflammation of WAT, constituting an important adipokines and triglycerides source which will be related with breast cancer development [52]. There are several adipokines secreted by adipose tissue that are implied with breast cancer [53]. Specially, increased leptin levels are related not only with breast cancer but also with obesity [54]. Leptin is the responsible for the mammary glands development and lactation, in addition to the breast cancer proliferation and invasion [55]. In fact, higher levels of leptin have been observed in women with breast cancer compared to healthy women. On the other hand, it has been described that adiponectin levels are inversely proportional to adiposity, exerting an inhibitory action on tumor growth and proliferation as well as stimulating apoptosis [56]. That is why lower levels of this adiponectin have been observed in patients with obesity [52]. Regarding insulin, obese and breast cancer women present higher circulating levels. Insulin induces proliferation of the breast cancer cells with ER+ by realizing growth factors that stimulate mitosis and inhibit apoptosis [57]. Finally, it should be noted that obese women with breast cancer have low levels of sex hormone-binding globulin (SHBG) [58]. This protein binds to sex steroids, regulating their bioavailability in the bloodstream. Therefore, this is the reason by which obese women with breast cancer have elevated levels of estrogen in their breast tissues.

While the principle supply of estrogen in premenopausal women is the ovarics, in postmenopausal women estrogen synthesis is located in peripheral tissues along with WAT (which include mammary glands) and endothelial tissue [59]. In this case, estrogens are synthesized by transformation of androgenic precursors of adrenal origin or biologically inactive estrogens. Adipose tissue from mammary glands is composed of fibroblasts and endothelial cells. Breast cancer risk is correlated to the increased amount of adipose tissue, particularly in undifferentiated fibroblasts, due to this tissue has high aromatase activity, responsible for stimulating the synthesis of estrogens, and its promoters [60]. In normal breast tissue there is a high concentration of inactive steroids and the expression and activity of EST tend to be increased. In contrast, in breast tumor tissue, aromatase, 17βHSD, and steroid sulfatase (STS) tend to be overexpressed while EST expression and activity is decreased, resulting in an accumulation of 17beta-estradiol in breast tumor tissues [61, 62].

Estrogens are necessary to the malignant epithelial cells' growth. These cells produce antiadipogenic cytokines (IL-6, IL-11 and TNF-α and PGE2), that increase the cAMP levels which stimulate the aromatase promoters, giving place an up-regulation of aromatase expression in the preadipocytes. This is the reason why there are a great number of estrogens in adipose tissue fibroblasts. Furthermore, the antiadipogenic cytokines are responsible for the inhibition of the adipogenic cytokines, PPARγ and C/EBPα, stopping the differentiation of preadipocytes into mature adipocytes [63]. All these processes are known as desmoplastic reaction [64].

3.2 Melatonin and desmoplastic reaction

Melatonin stimulates the adipogenic cytokines, peroxisome proliferator-activated receptor gamma (PPARγ) and CCAAT-enhancer-binding proteins (C/EBPα), promoting the differentiation of preadipocytes into mature adipocytes [65]. Besides, melatonin inhibits the expression of aromatase promoters lowering the estrogen circulating levels [64]. This hormone is able to inhibit cyclooxygenase activity, thus reducing PGE2 levels, and decreasing intracellular cAMP. This fact will inhibit the aromatase promoters in peritumoral fibroblasts, reducing the expression and activity of aromatase and, therefore, the local estrogen levels in breast tissue [66]. Finally, melatonin reduces the antiadipogenic cytokines production in malignant epithelial cells, being related this with the aromatase expression.

As already has been described in a previous section, melatonin acts as a SEEM and SERM, reducing the estradiol concentrations in tumors, and therefore reducing the risk of breast cancer [42, 43, 67, 68].

Finally, melatonin is associated with a reduction in the risk of obesity related to breast cancer because increases adiponectin secretion; inhibits aromatase expression; inhibits leptin levels; reduces blood glucose and insulin resistance; and decreases body fat mass [57].

4. Melatonin and the estrobolome in breast cancer

It is known that both changes in the production of melatonin (circadian disruption) and the imbalance in the composition of the microbiota (dysbiosis) produce alterations in estrogen levels, which is one of the main risk factors for the development of breast cancer. Therefore, since a relationship between circadian disruption and breast cancer and between dysbiosis and breast cancer have been described, here we claim to describe the link between gut microbiota, melatonin, and breast cancer.

Bacterial composition of estrobolome in turn is probably affected by different factors, which can exert selective pressures on bacterial populations and can cause an imbalance or dysbiosis, which increases the risk of breast cancer due to elevated levels of circulating estrogens in postmenopausal women [69]. Melatonin modulates the composition of the microbiota and suppresses pathogenic bacteria in the gut due through its antioxidant activities [70]. Additionally, significantly, enteric cells and gut microbiota produce large amounts of melatonin. Circadian disruption, caused by sleep deprivation or exposure to constant light, causes an alteration in the composition of intestinal bacteria (dysbiosis) and affects the levels of melatonin [70]. Some authors demonstrated that exogenous melatonin supplementation restores microbiota composition [71] by reducing oxidative stress and the inflammatory response by suppressing toll-like receptor 4 (TLR4) expression, suggesting that melatonin may interact directly with gut microbiota. Thus, since melatonin modulates microbiota composition, involved in the pathogenesis of various cancers, a link exists between melatonin, microbiota, and the pathogenesis of cancer caused by dysbiosis [70].

Regarding breast cancer, gut microbiome is fundamental for the regulation of steroid hormone metabolism. It is crucial in the development of hormone receptor-positive breast cancer, whose circulating estrogen levels are the most important risk factor. Alterations in the bacterial composition of the estrobolome favor bacteria with β-glucuronidase activity, which deconjugate estrogens, favoring their enterohepatic circulation, causing their reabsorption and increasing the total estrogen load, and therefore increasing the risk of breast cancer [72].

On the other hand, melatonin increases the expression and activity of EST and reduces the expression and activity of STS, increasing the concentration of conjugated estrogens (biologically inactive) that are excreted in the bile and reducing the amount of deconjugated (biologically active) estrogens [44]. Therefore, this neurohormone exerts an activity opposite to the β-glucuronidase activity of intestinal bacteria, reducing the number of estrogens and lowering the risk of developing breast cancer [21].

Apart from this effect, changes in the intestinal microbiota activate the kynurenine pathway, moving Trp away from the melatonergic pathway and reducing the amount of melatonin and thus increasing the risk of breast cancer. In addition, butyrate favors the melatonergic pathway, so a reduction in this SCFA will produce a decrease in melatonin, increasing the NAS/melatonin ratio. NAS activates TrkB, activating the PI3K/AKT, MAPK, and PLC/PKC pathways, which are involved in cancer cell survival, migration, invasion, and metastasis. Therefore, dysbiosis leads to lower concentrations of butyrate and melatonin, which can result in inflammation and an increase in estrogens in the bloodstream and, therefore, an increase in breast cancer risk [73].

5. Gut permeability, intestinal dysbiosis, and circadian disruption

Dysbiosis and circadian disturbances induce the appearance of various diseases, including cancer. These disorders are characterized by an increase in gut permeability, which allows the passage of compounds such as LPS that interact with the immune system, causing inflammatory gut diseases [74].

A diet rich in fats and sugars causes an imbalance in bacteria composition, favoring the appearance of pathologies that are further pronounced by the circadian disruption [74]. This kind of diet has been shown to increase the abundance of Firmicutes, Proteobacteria, and Verrucomicrobia, and decrease the abundance of Bacteroidetes [74]. This dysbiosis is associated with a reduction in SCFAs production (especially butyrate) and an increase in the LPS levels, inducing gut permeability. Butyrate is related to the maintenance of gut barrier and the increased natural killer cytotoxicity, allowing the removal of viruses and cancer cells [75].

Increase in intestinal permeability is related to a reduction of calcium absorption produced by a vitamin D decreased [76], which produces a reduction in intestinal motility. This situation will allow the transfer of LPS to the circulation, which will activate the CD14/TLR2/4/MD2 pathogen recognition system [77]. The activation of this complex activates the Nuclear Factor kappa-light-chain-enhancer of activated B cells (NFkβ), activating the inflammatory cytokines and thus triggering strong autoimmune inflammatory activity that will be associated with cancer [76, 77]. Melatonin reduces the levels of these proinflammatory cytokines and inhibits NFkβ, modulating inflammation and reducing permeability [75, 78]. Furthermore, melatonin is able to reduce permeability by preserving mitochondrial-function mechanism [79] and releasing acetylcholine in the vagus nerve, which activates α7nAChR in intestinal cells [75, 80]. Apart from this, melatonin inhibits NOD-like Receptor 3 (NLRP3) and NOD-like Receptor pyrin domain-containing-6 (NLRP6), decreasing permeability [77]. Butyrate may also act as NLRP3 inhibitor, behaving similarly to melatonin [73].

On the other hand, circadian disruption induces an increase in proinflammatory cytokines, causing the loosening of tight junctions in intestinal epithelial cells and also increasing permeability [75]. When circadian disruption occurs, a significant increase in de abundance of Firmicutes is observed and this abundance was even higher when this situation is combined with a diet rich in fats and sugars. In addition, an increase in Ruminococcus and Sporosarcina was observed, accompanied by a reduction in Desulfosporosinus and Desulfotomocalum. Alternatively, melatonin can restore microbiota composition, reducing Clostridiales abundance and increasing Lactobacillus [81]. It is important to highlight that when circadian disruption occurs, there is an increase in the pro-inflammatory bacteria Ruminococcus and a reduction in the antiinflammatory bacteria Lactobacillus, which is associated with the NFkβ inhibition. All this suggests that circadian disruption favors inflammation and permeability, which are characteristics of cancers [74].

6. Clinical trials and possible applications of melatonin in breast cancer treatment

Clinical trials suggest that melatonin, due to its antioxidant, immunomodulatory, antiestrogenic, proapoptotic, and antiproliferative properties [82], can have a protective effect when administered along with other treatments such as chemotherapy or radiotherapy in patients suffering from advanced solid tumors [83]. The most outstanding results have been particularly obtained in breast cancer. Melatonin is an antitumor agent that enhances the beneficial effects of chemotherapy and radiotherapy and, on the other hand, it protects against the side effects of these therapies [83].

Melatonin has been shown to have anticancer actions in both *in vivo* and *in vitro* models and has been shown to reduce estrogenic hormones responsible for the normal and pathological growth of the mammary gland. It interferes with the activation of the estrogen receptor and counteracts the effects of estrogen at the tumor cell level, behaving as a SERM. Currently, 22 clinical trials examining the therapeutic value of melatonin in breast cancer are listed on the ClinicalTrials.gov. database. 5 of them are focused on the relief of symptoms associated with the tumoral process. The remaining 17 studies examine the therapeutic effects of melatonin either alone (9 trials) or as an adjuvant therapy associated with metformin, vitamin D, fluorouracil, doxorubicin, or toremifene (6 trials) or as an adjuvant therapy associated with radiotherapy (2 trials) in women already diagnosed with breast cancer.

In vitro, it has been demonstrated that melatonin increases the sensitivity of breast cancer cells to the effects of tamoxifen and anti-aromatase treatments [84, 85]. Furthermore, melatonin can behave as a preventive agent for breast cancer. Hormone replacement therapy (HRT) and cancer are controversial. Some clinical trials demonstrate that breast cancer is related to women who receive HRT, while others demonstrate that it does not affect increasing breast cancer risk [86]. Melatonin administration to patients who received previously HRT reduces the possibility of breast cancer development [87]. On the other hand, melatonin is able to reduce the breast cancer risk associated with obesity because this hormone prevents obesity and reduces aromatase expression and activity, thereby reducing the estrogen levels in adipose tissue [88]. Breast cancer risk is also associated with the exposure to some environmental pollutants with estrogenic properties (xenoestrogens). In particular, melatonin has been studied to counteract the estrogenic effects induced by cadmium [41, 89, 90], being useful to women who work in environments with these chemical pollutants. Besides, melatonin supplement has been shown to prevent chronodisruption induced by the exposure to light at night in women who work at night [91, 92].

Finally, melatonin has been shown to behave as an adjuvant agent that prevents the side effects of breast cancer treatments. In particular, melatonin has been studied for the improvement of sleep and life quality [93]. A prospective phase II trial showed that melatonin improves quality of sleep and life, social functions, reduces fatigue, and increases clock genes expression [93]. Another randomized, placebo-controlled, and double-blind clinical trial in postmenopausal breast cancer survivors showed that melatonin improved the quality of sleep but had no effect on hot flashes [94]. Melatonin as an adjuvant of anti-aromatase therapies prevents the osteoporosis induced by these treatments since this hormone promotes osteoblasts proliferation [95].

Besides, melatonin has been studied as the treatment of depressive symptoms and anxiety [96]. In particular, a study on women undergoing breast cancer surgery showed that melatonin reduced the risk of depressive symptoms [96]. Patients treated not only with tamoxifen but also con melatonin, felt an improvement in anxiety, asthenia, and symptoms of depression in comparison with those treated with tamoxifen alone [97].

In addition, melatonin is described as the prevention of breast radiation dermatitis [98]. Topical applications of melatonin emulsions to the management of skin toxicity during radiotherapy have been proposed [99]. In this sense, A phase II, prospective, double-blind randomized trial was designed to evaluate the efficacy of melatonin-containing cream (twice daily) in breast cancer patients during radiation treatment. In conclusion, patients in the melatonin group experimented a significantly reduced radiation dermatitis compared to those women receiving placebo [98].

On the other hand, melatonin is able to decrease the toxicity and increase the efficacy of chemotherapy [100]. It has been demonstrated that melatonin may protect patients against side effects such as stomatitis, asthenia, cardiotoxicity, and neurotoxicity caused by chemotherapy [101]. Melatonin reduces the hepatotoxicity induced by anti-aromatase therapies, such as letrozole [33]. Besides, melatonin decreases damage caused for chemotherapy drugs in blood cells [102]. In breast, lung, and gastrointestinal cancer patients, melatonin preserved against thrombocytopenia, stomatitis, asthenia, and neuropathy [103]. A hybrid compound of melatonin and tamoxifen has been patented (US8785501) to combine antiestrogenic properties of these compounds and reduce the side effects of tamoxifen, reducing the hyperproliferation uterine risk [104, 105]. Previous studies have also demonstrated that the percentage of 1-year survival in patients with advanced non-small-cell lung cancer treated with cisplatin and melatonin and in breast cancer treated with tamoxifen and melatonin increased in comparison with patients treated only with chemotherapy [97].

Despite the promising experimental results about the radioprotective role of melatonin, few clinical trials to verify the therapeutic usefulness of melatonin in humans have been conducted. In this sense, a preliminary study suggests that adjuvant melatonin plus radiotherapy may prolong the 1-year survival rate and improve the quality of life of patients affected by untreatable glioblastoma [106].

Thus, it exists a plethora of applications of melatonin, which could be a promising future target of study in the pathology of breast cancer.

7. Conclusions

Breast cancer is a multifactorial disease. However, an explanation for the mechanism, which triggers this pathology remains unclear, and there lacks a hypothesis that can link all the mechanisms together. Over the years, researchers have studied the enormous range of biological activities of melatonin and its potential applications, including its effects as anticancer molecule. Recently, this indolamine has been described as a promising adjuvant in ER breast cancer prevention and treatment because of its antiestrogenic properties.

Herein we have proposed that a link between gut microbiota and melatonin levels exists, as well as between dysbiosis and circadian disruption, leading to an increase in the circulation of estrogen levels that is able to induce the development of breast cancer. On the other hand, butyrate is an SCFA synthesized by the intestinal microbiota that stimulates the melatonergic pathway by promoting the production of melatonin. Nevertheless, proinflammatory cytokines, stress, and diet factors stimulate the kynurenine pathway, moving Trp away from melatonergic pathway. This situation contributes to reducing melatonin levels and favoring NAS levels, increasing the NAS/melatonin ratio in breast cancer patients. It is important to highlight that NAS is implicated in survival, proliferation, and metastasis of breast cancer cells. In addition, this generates changes in gut microbiome and intestinal permeability caused by butyrate reduction and LPS levels increasing, inducing the inflammatory response, and decreasing melatonin production. All the foregoing contribute to breast cancer development.

Regarding changes in estrobolome composition as well as chronodisruption, favor the presence of deconjugated state of estrogens, which are the active form that increases breast cancer risk. We described the opposite action that melatonin exerts, unlike gut microbiome-derived β-glucuronidase activity. Melatonin is able to reduce the expression and activity of enzymes important in the biosynthesis of estrogens, reducing the estrogens levels and preventing breast cancer appearance.

On the other hand, melatonin regulates the desmoplastic reaction inducing the differentiation of preadipocytes into mature adipocytes, which do not express aromatase, lowering levels of estrogens and then reducing breast cancer risk. Melatonin achieves this differentiation through the stimulation of adipogenic cytokines (PPARγ and C/EBPα) and the inhibition of antiadipogenic cytokines (TNFα, IL-6, IL-11).

Although many in vitro and in vivo studies have been described, more clinical trials will be needed to describe the sensitizing properties of melatonin to the different treatments used to treat breast cancer, as well as to avoid their side effects. In addition, it will be important to explore the relationship between melatonin and the intestinal microbiota, since measuring the levels of this hormone together with the determination of the composition of the estrobolome of patients with breast cancer could constitute a promising tool for the development of biomarkers that help predict the development of breast cancer earlier. In conclusion, it will be crucial to maintain adequate levels of melatonin and a balanced composition of the microbiota to avoid developing breast cancer.

Acknowledgements

This work was funded in part by PE-0106-2019 from the Consejería de Salud de la Junta de Andalucía, C19047-2018 from Fundación Unicaja and UMA18-FEDERJA-042 from UMA-FEDER & ALIANZA MIXTA ANDALUCÍA-ROCHE. María Isabel Queipo Ortuño is recipient of a "Miguel Servet Type II" program (CPI13/00003) from ISCIII, co-funded by the Fondo Europeo de Desarrollo Regional-FEDER, Madrid, Spain and also belongs to the regional "Nicolas Monardes" research program of the Consejería de Salud (C-0030-2018, Junta de Andalucía, Spain. Alicia González González is recipient of a postdoctoral grant Margarita Salas (RMS-08) from European Union-NextGenerationEU, Spanish Ministry of Universities and Recovery Transformation and Resilience Plan, through a call from University of Cantabria. Aurora Laborda Illanes is recipient of a predoctoral grant, PFIS-ISCIII (FI19-00112), co-funded by the Fondo Social Europeo (FSE). Lidia Sanchez Alcoholado is recipient of a predoctoral grant (PE-0106-2019) from the Consejería de Salud y Familia (co-funded by the

Fondo Europeo de Desarrollo Regional-FEDER, Andalucía, Spain). Daniel Castellano Castillo is recipient of a postdoctoral grant Sara Borrell (CD21/00164) from Instituto de Salud Carlos III.

Conflict of interest

The authors declare no conflict of interest.

Author details

Alicia González-González[1,2,3]*, Aurora Laborda-Illanes[3], Soukaina Boutriq[3], Lidia Sánchez-Alcoholado[3], Daniel Castellano-Castillo[3], Isaac Plaza-Andrades[3], Jesús Peralta-Linero[3] and María Isabel Queipo-Ortuño[3,4]

1 Faculty of Medicine, Department of Medicine and Pediatrics, University of Malaga, Malaga, Spain

2 Faculty of Medicine, Pharmacology, University of Cantabria and Valdecilla Health Research Institute (IDIVAL), Santander, Spain

3 Regional and Virgen de la Victoria University Hospitals, Intercenter Medical Oncology Clinical Management Unit, Malaga Biomedical Research Institute (IBIMA)-CIMES-UMA, Malaga, Spain

4 Faculty of Medicine, Department of Surgical Specialties, Biochemical and Immunology, University of Málaga, Malaga, Spain

*Address all correspondence to: alicia.gonzalez@ibima.eu

References

[1] Breast Cancer Prevention (PDQ®)–Patient Version - National Cancer Institute [Internet]. 2021 [citado 26 de abril de 2022]. Disponible en: https://www.cancer.gov/types/breast/patient/breast-prevention-pdq

[2] Mediavilla MD, Sanchez-Barcelo EJ, Tan DX, Manchester L, Reiter RJ. Basic mechanisms involved in the anti-cancer effects of melatonin. Current Medicinal Chemistry. 2010;**17**(36):4462-4481

[3] Acuña-Castroviejo D, Escames G, Venegas C, Díaz-Casado ME, Lima-Cabello E, López LC, et al. Extrapineal melatonin: Sources, regulation, and potential functions. Cellular and Molecular Life Sciences. 2014;**71**(16):2997-3025

[4] Li Y, Hao Y, Fan F, Zhang B. The Role of Microbiome in Insomnia, Circadian Disturbance and Depression. Front Psychiatry. 2018;**9**:669

[5] Rosiak J, Zawilska JB. 14-3-3 proteins--a role in the regulation of melatonin biosynthesis. Postepy Biochemii. 2006;**52**(1):35-41

[6] Amaral FG, do, Cipolla-Neto J. A brief review about melatonin, a pineal hormone. Architecture Endocrinology Metabolism. 2018;**62**(4):472-479

[7] Badawy AAB. Kynurenine pathway and human systems. Experimental Gerontology. 2020;**129**:110770

[8] Chen Y, Guillemin G. The kynurenine pathway [internet]. Amyotrophic Lateral Sclerosis. IntechOpen, London, UK; 2012 [citado 11 de abril de 2022]. Disponible en: https://www.intechopen.com/chapters/26541

[9] Cervantes GIV, OlascoagaArellano NK, Ortega DR, Ramiro AS, Esquivel DFG, Ríos C, et al. Role of kynurenine pathway in glioblastoma [internet]. In: Mechanisms of Neuroinflammation. London, UK: IntechOpen; 2017 [citado 11 de abril de 2022]. Disponible en: https://www.intechopen.com/chapters/55661

[10] Badawy AAB. Kynurenine pathway of tryptophan metabolism: Regulatory and functional aspects. International Journal of Tryptophane Research. 2017;**10**:1178646917691938

[11] Al-Dhfyan A, Alhoshani A, Korashy HM. Aryl hydrocarbon receptor/cytochrome P450 1A1 pathway mediates breast cancer stem cells expansion through PTEN inhibition and β-catenin and Akt activation. Molecular Cancer. 2017;**16**(1):14

[12] Asghar K, Loya A, Rana IA, Tahseen M, Ishaq M, Farooq A, et al. Indoleamine 2,3-dioxygenase expression and overall survival in patients diagnosed with breast cancer in Pakistan. Cancer Management and Research. 2019;**11**:475-481

[13] Anderson G. Breast cancer: Occluded role of mitochondria N-acetylserotonin/melatonin ratio in co-ordinating pathophysiology. Biochemical Pharmacology. 2019;**168**:259-268

[14] Zhai L, Dey M, Lauing KL, Gritsina G, Kaur R, Lukas RV, et al. The kynurenine to tryptophan ratio as a prognostic tool for glioblastoma patients enrolling in immunotherapy. Journal of Clinical Neuroscience. 2015;**22**(12):1964-1968

[15] Ye Z, Yue L, Shi J, Shao M, Wu T. Role of IDO and TDO in cancers and

related diseases and the therapeutic implications. Journal of Cancer. 2019;**10**(12):2771-2782

[16] Muller AJ, DuHadaway JB, Donover PS, Sutanto-Ward E, Prendergast GC. Inhibition of indoleamine 2,3-dioxygenase, an immunoregulatory target of the cancer suppression gene Bin1, potentiates cancer chemotherapy. Nature Medicine. 2005;**11**(3):312-319

[17] Bjørn J. Peptide Vaccination in Combination With Either Ipilimumab or Vemurafenib for the Treatment of Patients With Unresectable Stage III or IV Malignant Melanoma A Phase I Study (First in Man) [Internet]. clinicaltrials.gov. 2014 [citado 17 de abril de 2022]. Report No.: NCT02077114. Disponible en: https://clinicaltrials.gov/ct2/show/NCT02077114

[18] Incyte Corporation. A Randomized, Open-Label, Phase 2 Study of the IDO Inhibitor Epacadostat Versus Tamoxifen for Subjects With Biochemical-Recurrent-Only Epithelial Ovarian Cancer, Primary Peritoneal Carcinoma, or Fallopian Tube Cancer Following Complete Remission With First-Line Chemotherapy [Internet]. clinicaltrials.gov. 2019 [citado 17 de abril de 2022]. Report No.: NCT01685255. Disponible en: https://clinicaltrials.gov/ct2/show/NCT01685255

[19] Iversen TZ, Engell-Noerregaard L, Ellebaek E, Andersen R, Larsen SK, Bjoern J, et al. Long-lasting disease stabilization in the absence of toxicity in metastatic lung cancer patients vaccinated with an epitope derived from indoleamine 2,3 dioxygenase. Clinical Cancer Research. 2014;**20**(1):221-232

[20] Vacchelli E, Aranda F, Eggermont A, Sautès-Fridman C, Tartour E, Kennedy EP, et al. Trial watch: IDO inhibitors in cancer therapy. Oncoimmunology. 2014;**3**(10):e957994

[21] Laborda-Illanes A, Sánchez-Alcoholado L, Boutriq S, Plaza-Andrades I, Peralta-Linero J, Alba E, et al. A new paradigm in the relationship between melatonin and breast cancer: Gut microbiota identified as a potential regulatory agent. Cancers. 2021;**13**(13):3141

[22] Kiefer T, Ram PT, Yuan L, Hill SM. Melatonin inhibits estrogen receptor transactivation and cAMP levels in breast cancer cells. Breast Cancer Research and Treatment. 2002;**71**(1):37-45

[23] Aronica SM, Kraus WL, Katzenellenbogen BS. Estrogen action via the cAMP signaling pathway: Stimulation of adenylate cyclase and cAMP-regulated gene transcription. Proceedings of the National Academy of Sciences of the United States of America. 1994;**91**(18):8517-8521

[24] García Pedrero JM, Del Rio B, Martínez-Campa C, Muramatsu M, Lazo PS, Ramos S. Calmodulin is a selective modulator of estrogen receptors. Molecular Endocrinology. 2002;**16**(5):947-960

[25] del Río B, García Pedrero JM, Martínez-Campa C, Zuazua P, Lazo PS, Ramos S. Melatonin, an endogenous-specific inhibitor of estrogen receptor alpha via calmodulin. The Journal of Biological Chemistry. 2004;**279**(37):38294-38302

[26] Dong C, Yuan L, Dai J, Lai L, Mao L, Xiang S, et al. Melatonin inhibits mitogenic cross-talk between retinoic acid-related orphan receptor alpha (RORalpha) and ERalpha in MCF-7 human breast cancer cells. Steroids. 2010;**75**(12):944-951

[27] Allegra M, Reiter RJ, Tan DX, Gentile C, Tesoriere L, Livrea MA. The chemistry of melatonin's interaction

with reactive species. Journal of Pineal Research. 2003;**34**(1):1-10

[28] Cos S, Sánchez-Barceló EJ. Melatonin and mammary pathological growth. Frontiers in Neuroendocrinology. 2000;**21**(2):133-170

[29] Sainz R, Mayo J, Rodriguez C, Tan D, López-Burillo S, Reiter RJ. Melatonin and cell death: Differential actions on apoptosis in normal and cancer cells. Cellular and molecular life sciences, 2003;**60**(7):1407-26

[30] Reiter RJ, Rosales-Corral SA, Tan DX, Acuna-Castroviejo D, Qin L, Yang SF, et al. Melatonin, a full service anti-cancer agent: Inhibition of initiation, progression and metastasis. International Journal of Molecular Sciences. 2017;**18**(4):E843

[31] Galano A, Tan DX, Reiter RJ. Melatonin as a natural ally against oxidative stress: A physicochemical examination. Journal of Pineal Research. 2011;**51**(1):1-16

[32] Kelleher FC, Rao A, Maguire A. Circadian molecular clocks and cancer. Cancer Letters. 2014;**342**(1):9-18

[33] Hill SM, Belancio VP, Dauchy RT, Xiang S, Brimer S, Mao L, et al. Melatonin: An inhibitor of breast cancer. Endocrine-Related Cancer. 2015;**22**(3):R183-R204

[34] Cos S, Recio J, Sánchez-Barceló EJ. Modulation of the length of the cell cycle time of MCF-7 human breast cancer cells by melatonin. Life Sciences. 1996;**58**(9):811-816

[35] Cos S, Blask DE, Lemus-Wilson A, Hill AB. Effects of melatonin on the cell cycle kinetics and «estrogen-rescue» of MCF-7 human breast cancer cells in culture. Journal of Pineal Research. 1991;**10**(1):36-42

[36] Cui P, Luo Z, Zhang H, Su Y, Li A, Li H, et al. Effect and mechanism of melatonin's action on the proliferation of human umbilical vein endothelial cells. Journal of Pineal Research. 2006;**41**(4):358-362

[37] Alvarez-García V, González A, Alonso-González C, Martínez-Campa C, Cos S. Antiangiogenic effects of melatonin in endothelial cell cultures. Microvascular Research. 2013;**87**:25-33

[38] Mao L, Yuan L, Slakey LM, Jones FE, Burow ME, Hill SM. Inhibition of breast cancer cell invasion by melatonin is mediated through regulation of the p38 mitogen-activated protein kinase signaling pathway. Breast Cancer Research. 2010;**12**(6):R107

[39] Maroufi NF, Ashouri N, Mortezania Z, Ashoori Z, Vahedian V, Amirzadeh-Iranaq MT, et al. The potential therapeutic effects of melatonin on breast cancer: An invasion and metastasis inhibitor. Pathology, Research and Practice. 2020;**216**(10):153226

[40] Leon-Blanco MM, Guerrero JM, Reiter RJ, Calvo JR, Pozo D. Melatonin inhibits telomerase activity in the MCF-7 tumor cell line both in vivo and in vitro. Journal of Pineal Research. 2003;**35**(3):204-211

[41] Martínez-Campa CM, Alonso-González C, Mediavilla MD, Cos S, González A, Sanchez-Barcelo EJ. Melatonin down-regulates hTERT expression induced by either natural estrogens (17beta-estradiol) or metalloestrogens (cadmium) in MCF-7 human breast cancer cells. Cancer Letters. 2008;**268**(2):272-277

[42] Cos S, González A, Martínez-Campa C, Mediavilla MD, Alonso-González C, Sánchez-Barceló EJ. Estrogen-signaling pathway: A link

between breast cancer and melatonin oncostatic actions. Cancer Detection and Prevention. 2006;**30**(2):118-128

[43] Cos S, González A, Martínez-Campa C, Mediavilla MD, Alonso-González C, Sánchez-Barceló EJ. Melatonin as a selective estrogen enzyme modulator. Current Cancer Drug Targets. 2008;**8**(8):691-702

[44] Martínez-Campa C, González A, Mediavilla MD, Alonso-González C, Alvarez-García V, Sánchez-Barceló EJ, et al. Melatonin inhibits aromatase promoter expression by regulating cyclooxygenases expression and activity in breast cancer cells. British Journal of Cancer. 2009;**101**(9):1613-1619

[45] Gonzalez A, Cos S, Martinez-Campa C, Alonso-Gonzalez C, Sanchez-Mateos S, Mediavilla MD, et al. Selective estrogen enzyme modulator actions of melatonin in human breast cancer cells. Journal of Pineal Research. 2008;**45**(1):86-92

[46] Cohen M, Lippman M, Chabner B. Role of pineal gland in aetiology and treatment of breast cancer. Lancet. 1978;**2**(8094):814-816

[47] Danforth DN, Tamarkin L, Mulvihill JJ, Bagley CS, Lippman ME. Plasma melatonin and the hormone-dependency of human breast cancer. Journal of Clinical Oncology. 1985;**3**(7):941-948

[48] Skene DJ, Bojkowski CJ, Currie JE, Wright J, Boulter PS, Arendt J. 6-sulphatoxymelatonin production in breast cancer patients. Journal of Pineal Research. 1990;**8**(3):269-276

[49] Orendáš P, Kubatka P, Bojková B, Kassayová M, Kajo K, Výbohová D, et al. Melatonin potentiates the anti-tumour effect of pravastatin in rat mammary gland carcinoma model. International Journal of Experimental Pathology. 2014;**95**(6):401-410

[50] Cos S, Bardasano JL, Mediavilla MD, Sánchez Barceló EJ. Pineal gland in rats with 7,12-dimethylbenz(a)anthracene-induced mammary tumors subjected to manipulations known as enhancers of pineal actions. Histology and Histopathology. 1989;**4**(2):235-239

[51] Lissoni P. Biochemotherapy with standard chemotherapies plus the pineal hormone melatonin in the treatment of advanced solid neoplasms. Pathology Biology (Paris). 2007;**55**(3-4):201-204

[52] Macis D, Guerrieri-Gonzaga A, Gandini S. Circulating adiponectin and breast cancer risk: A systematic review and meta-analysis. International Journal of Epidemiology. 2014;**43**(4):1226-1236

[53] Gui Y, Pan Q, Chen X, Xu S, Luo X, Chen L. The association between obesity related adipokines and risk of breast cancer: A meta-analysis. Oncotarget. 2017;**8**(43):75389-75399

[54] Smith-Kirwin SM, O'Connor DM, De Johnston J, Lancey ED, Hassink SG, Funanage VL. Leptin expression in human mammary epithelial cells and breast milk. The Journal of Clinical Endocrinology and Metabolism. 1998;**83**(5):1810-1813

[55] Karaduman M, Bilici A, Ozet A, Sengul A, Musabak U, Alomeroglu M. Tissue leptin levels in patients with breast cancer. Journal of BUON. 2010;**15**(2):369-372

[56] Yunusova NV, Kondakova IV, Kolomiets LA, Afanas'ev SG, Chernyshova AL, Kudryavtsev IV, et al. Molecular targets for the therapy of cancer associated with metabolic syndrome (transcription and growth factors). Asia-Pacific Journal of Clinical Oncology. 2018;**14**(3):134-140

[57] González-González A, Mediavilla MD, Sánchez-Barceló EJ. Melatonin: A molecule for reducing breast cancer risk. Molecules. 2018;**23**(2):336

[58] Simó R, Sáez-López C, Barbosa-Desongles A, Hernández C, Selva DM. Novel insights in SHBG regulation and clinical implications. Trends in Endocrinology and Metabolism. 2015;**26**(7):376-383

[59] Martínez-Chacón G, Brown KA, Docanto MM, Kumar H, Salminen S, Saarinen N, et al. IL-10 suppresses TNF-α-induced expression of human aromatase gene in mammary adipose tissue. The FASEB Journal. 2018;**32**(6):3361-3370

[60] Lønning PE, Helle H, Duong NK, Ekse D, Aas T, Geisler J. Tissue estradiol is selectively elevated in receptor positive breast cancers while tumour estrone is reduced independent of receptor status. The Journal of Steroid Biochemistry and Molecular Biology. 2009;**117**(1-3):31-41

[61] Pasqualini JR, Chetrite GS. Recent insight on the control of enzymes involved in estrogen formation and transformation in human breast cancer. The Journal of Steroid Biochemistry and Molecular Biology. 2005;**93**(2):221-236

[62] Suzuki T, Miki Y, Nakamura Y, Moriya T, Ito K, Ohuchi N, et al. Sex steroid-producing enzymes in human breast cancer. Endocrine-Related Cancer. 2005;**12**(4):701-720

[63] Rybinska I, Agresti R, Trapani A, Tagliabue E, Triulzi T. Adipocytes in breast cancer, the thick and the thin. Cell. 2020;**9**(3):560

[64] Cos S, Alvarez-García V, González A, Alonso-González C, Martínez-Campa C. Melatonin modulation of crosstalk among malignant epithelial, endothelial and adipose cells in breast cancer (review). Oncology Letters. 2014;**8**(2):487-492

[65] González A, Alvarez-García V, Martínez-Campa C, Alonso-González C, Cos S. Melatonin promotes differentiation of 3T3-L1 fibroblasts. Journal of Pineal Research. 2012;**52**(1):12-20

[66] Zhao Y, Agarwal VR, Mendelson CR, Simpson ER. Estrogen biosynthesis proximal to a breast tumor is stimulated by PGE2 via cyclic AMP, leading to activation of promoter II of the CYP19 (aromatase) gene. Endocrinology. 1996;**137**(12):5739-5742

[67] Cos S, Martínez-Campa C, Mediavilla MD, Sánchez-Barceló EJ. Melatonin modulates aromatase activity in MCF-7 human breast cancer cells. Journal of Pineal Research. 2005;**38**(2):136-142

[68] González A, Alvarez-García V, Martínez-Campa C, Mediavilla MD, Alonso-González C, Sánchez-Barceló EJ, et al. In vivo inhibition of the estrogen sulfatase enzyme and growth of DMBA-induced mammary tumors by melatonin. Current Cancer Drug Targets. 2010;**10**(3):279-286

[69] Kwa M, Plottel CS, Blaser MJ, Adams S. The intestinal microbiome and estrogen receptor-positive female breast cancer. Journal of the National Cancer Institute. 2016;**108**(8):djw029

[70] Bonmati-Carrion MA, Tomas-Loba A. Melatonin and cancer: A polyhedral network where the source matters. Antioxidants (Basel). 2021;**10**(2):210

[71] Ren W, Wang P, Yan J, Liu G, Zeng B, Hussain T, et al. Melatonin alleviates

weanling stress in mice: Involvement of intestinal microbiota. Journal of Pineal Research. 2018;**64**(2)

[72] Parida S, Sharma D. The microbiome–estrogen connection and breast cancer risk. Cell. 2019;**8**(12):1642

[73] Anderson G. Gut dysbiosis dysregulates central and systemic homeostasis via decreased me latonin and suboptimal mitochondria functioning: Pathoetiological and pathophysiological implications. Melatonin Research. 2019;**2**:70-85

[74] Voigt RM, Forsyth CB, Green SJ, Mutlu E, Engen P, Vitaterna MH, et al. Circadian disorganization alters intestinal microbiota. PLoS One. 2014;**9**(5):e97500

[75] Anderson G, Reiter RJ. COVID-19 pathophysiology: Interactions of gut microbiome, melatonin, vitamin D, stress, kynurenine and the alpha 7 nicotinic receptor: Treatment implications. Melatonin Research. 2020;**3**(3):322-345

[76] Ghareghani M, Reiter RJ, Zibara K, Farhadi N. Latitude, vitamin D, melatonin, and gut microbiota act in concert to initiate multiple sclerosis: A new mechanistic pathway. Frontiers in Immunology. 2018;**9**:2484

[77] Anderson G, Maes M. The gut–brain axis: The role of melatonin in linking psychiatric, inflammatory and neurodegenerative conditions. Advances In Integrative Medicine. 2015;**2**:31-37

[78] Mannino G, Caradonna F, Cruciata I, Lauria A, Perrone A, Gentile C. Melatonin reduces inflammatory response in human intestinal epithelial cells stimulated by interleukin-1β. Journal of Pineal Research. 2019;**67**(3):e12598

[79] Mei Q, Diao L, Xu J, ming, Liu X chang, Jin J. A protective effect of melatonin on intestinal permeability is induced by diclofenac via regulation of mitochondrial function in mice. Acta Pharmacologica Sinica. 2011;**32**(4):495-502

[80] Gao J, Xu K, Liu H, Liu G, Bai M, Peng C, et al. Impact of the gut microbiota on intestinal immunity mediated by tryptophan metabolism. Frontiers in Cellular and Infection Microbiology. 2018;**8**:13

[81] Jing Y, Yang D, Bai F, Zhang C, Qin C, Li D, et al. Melatonin treatment alleviates spinal cord injury-induced gut Dysbiosis in mice. Journal of Neurotrauma. 2019;**36**(18):2646-2664

[82] Dakshayani KB, Subramanian P, Manivasagam T, Essa MM, Manoharan S. Melatonin modulates the oxidant-antioxidant imbalance during N-nitrosodiethylamine induced hepatocarcinogenesis in rats. Journal of Pharmacy & Pharmaceutical Sciences. 2005;**8**(2):316-321

[83] Alonso-Gonzalez C, González A, Cos S, González-González A, Menéndez-Menéndez J, Martinez-Campa C. Melatonin as modulator of radiosensibility and chemosensibility in cancer. Pineal Gland: Research Advances and Clinical Challenges. 2017;**11**:291-326

[84] Wilson ST, Blask DE, Lemus-Wilson AM. Melatonin augments the sensitivity of MCF-7 human breast cancer cells to tamoxifen in vitro. The Journal of Clinical Endocrinology and Metabolism. 1992;**75**(2):669-670

[85] Martínez-Campa C, González A, Mediavilla MD, Alonso-González C, Sánchez-Barceló EJ, Cos S. Melatonin enhances the inhibitory effect of

aminoglutethimide on aromatase activity in MCF-7 human breast cancer cells. Breast Cancer Research and Treatment. 2005;**94**(3):249-254

[86] Lobo RA. Hormone-replacement therapy: Current thinking. Nature Reviews. Endocrinology. 2017;**13**(4):220-231

[87] Witt-Enderby PA, Davis VL. Combination Hormone Replacement Therapy (HRT) and Melatonin to Prevent and Treat Mammary Cancer [Internet]. US8618083B2. 2013 [citado 31 de marzo de 2021]. Disponible en: https://patents.google.com/patent/US8618083B2/en?oq=US8618083

[88] Nduhirabandi F, Du Toit EF, Blackhurst D, Marais D, Lochner A. Chronic melatonin consumption prevents obesity-related metabolic abnormalities and protects the heart against myocardial ischemia and reperfusion injury in a prediabetic model of diet-induced obesity. Journal of Pineal Research. 2011;**50**(2):171-182

[89] Alonso-González C, González A, Mazarrasa O, Güezmes A, Sánchez-Mateos S, Martínez-Campa C, et al. Melatonin prevents the estrogenic effects of sub-chronic administration of cadmium on mice mammary glands and uterus. Journal of Pineal Research. 2007;**42**(4):403-410

[90] Alonso-Gonzalez C, Mediavilla D, Martinez-Campa C, Gonzalez A, Cos S, Sanchez-Barcelo EJ. Melatonin modulates the cadmium-induced expression of MT-2 and MT-1 metallothioneins in three lines of human tumor cells (MCF-7, MDA-MB-231 and HeLa). Toxicology Letters. 2008;**181**(3):190-195

[91] Hansen J. Night shift work and risk of breast cancer. Current Environment Health Reports. 2017;**4**(3):325-339

[92] Wu J, Dauchy RT, Tirrell PC, Wu SS, Lynch DT, Jitawatanarat P, et al. Light at night activates IGF-1R/PDK1 signaling and accelerates tumor growth in human breast cancer xenografts. Cancer Research. 2011;**71**(7):2622-2631

[93] Innominato PF, Lim AS, Palesh O, Clemons M, Trudeau M, Eisen A, et al. The effect of melatonin on sleep and quality of life in patients with advanced breast cancer. Supportive Care in Cancer. 2016;**24**(3):1097-1105

[94] Chen WY, Giobbie-Hurder A, Gantman K, Savoie J, Scheib R, Parker LM, et al. A randomized, placebo-controlled trial of melatonin on breast cancer survivors: Impact on sleep, mood, and hot flashes. Breast Cancer Research and Treatment. 2014;**145**(2):381-388

[95] Maria S, Witt-Enderby PA. Melatonin effects on bone: Potential use for the prevention and treatment for osteopenia, osteoporosis, and periodontal disease and for use in bone-grafting procedures. Journal of Pineal Research. 2014;**56**(2):115-125

[96] Hansen MV, Andersen LT, Madsen MT, Hageman I, Rasmussen LS, Bokmand S, et al. Effect of melatonin on depressive symptoms and anxiety in patients undergoing breast cancer surgery: A randomized, double-blind, placebo-controlled trial. Breast Cancer Research and Treatment. 2014;**145**(3):683-695

[97] Lissoni P, Ardizzoia A, Barni S, Brivio F, Tisi E, Rovelli F, et al. Efficacy and tolerability of cancer neuroimmunotherapy with subcutaneous low-dose interleukin-2 and the pineal hormone melatonin - a progress report of 200 patients with advanced solid neoplasms. Oncology Reports. 1995;**2**(6):1063-1068

[98] Ben-David MA, Elkayam R, Gelernter I, Pfeffer RM. Melatonin for prevention of breast radiation dermatitis: A phase II, prospective, double-blind randomized trial. The Israel Medical Association Journal. 2016;**18**(3-4):188-192

[99] Vasin MV, Ushakov IB, Kovtun VY, Komarova SN, Semenova LA. Effect of melatonin, ascorbic acid, and succinic acid on the cumulative toxic effect of repeated treatment with gammafos (amifostine). Bulletin of Experimental Biology and Medicine. 2004;**137**(5):450-452

[100] Lissoni P, Barni S, Mandalà M, Ardizzoia A, Paolorossi F, Vaghi M, et al. Decreased toxicity and increased efficacy of cancer chemotherapy using the pineal hormone melatonin in metastatic solid tumour patients with poor clinical status. European Journal of Cancer. 1999;**35**(12):1688-1692

[101] Kim C, Kim N, Joo H, Youm JB, Park WS, Cuong DV, et al. Modulation by melatonin of the cardiotoxic and antitumor activities of adriamycin. Journal of Cardiovascular Pharmacology. 2005;**46**(2):200-210

[102] Vijayalaxmi TCR, Reiter RJ, Herman TS. Melatonin: From basic research to cancer treatment clinics. Journal of Clinical Oncology. 2002;**20**(10):2575-2601

[103] Lissoni P, Tancini G, Barni S, Paolorossi F, Ardizzoia A, Conti A, et al. Treatment of cancer chemotherapy-induced toxicity with the pineal hormone melatonin. Support Care Cancer. 1997;**5**(2):126-129

[104] Witt-Enderby PA, Davis VL, Lapinsky D. Anti-Cancer Tamoxifen-Melatonin Hybrid Ligand [Internet]. US8785501B2. 2014. [citado 31 de marzo de 2021]. Disponible en: https://patents.google.com/patent/US8785501B2/en

[105] Hasan M, Leak RK, Stratford RE, Zlotos DP, Witt-Enderby PA. Drug conjugates-an emerging approach to treat breast cancer. Pharmacology Research & Perspectives. 2018;**6**(4):e00417

[106] Lissoni P, Meregalli S, Nosetto L, Barni S, Tancini G, Fossati V, et al. Increased survival time in brain glioblastomas by a radioneuroendocrine strategy with radiotherapy plus melatonin compared to radiotherapy alone. Oncology. 1996;**53**(1):43-46

Chapter 5

Melatonin in Cardiovascular Diseases

Hülya Kara and Adem Kara

Abstract

Melatonin is an endocrine product released from the gland known as the pineal gland and is predominantly secreted during the night. Light exerts an inhibitory effect on melatonin secretion in the pineal gland. The suprachiasmatic nucleus controls pineal melatonin synthesis and its release *via* the peripheral sympathetic nervous system, which includes synapses in the intermediolateral cell column of the thoracic cord and its projection toward the superior cervical ganglia. Melatonin regulates many physiological functions in the body through membrane receptors and nuclear binding sites. In a chick study, the presence of melatonin receptors in cardiomyocytes was reported and, in another study, MT1 and MT2 membrane receptors were identified in left ventricular cardiomyocytes of the human heart. For this reason, it is suggested that melatonin has some regulatory effects on the cardiovascular system. Ischemic heart disease and myocardial infarctions are the main cause of cardiovascular death. Studies have shown that melatonin applications reduce the amount of blood cholesterol, LDL, and triglyceride and increase the amount of HDL. In light of these data, it can be said that melatonin is an important cardiovascular system protector. In this chapter, the protective effects and mechanisms of melatonin on the cardiovascular system will be discussed.

Keywords: melatonin, cardiovascular diseases, heart, antioxidant, anti-inflammatory

1. Introduction

Melatonin [N-acetyl-5-methoxytryptamine] is a neuroendocrine hormone and was firstly isolated from the bovine pineal gland in 1958 by Lerner et al. [1]. The pineal gland is originating from the prosencephalon and was first identified by Herophilus in 325–280 BC. Photic data is received by photoreceptors in the retina and transmitted to the superior cervical ganglion via sympathetic preganglionic adrenergic neurons. Melatonin is synthesized from tryptophan through a number of enzymatic reactions in pinealocytes [2]. Melatonin secretion is regulated by the day/night events. In addition, while norepinephrine stimulates beta1-adrenoreceptors synthesis and secretion of melatonin, stimulation of alpha1-adrenoreceptors increases the reaction [3, 4]. While melatonin is mainly secreted from the pineal gland, melatonin is also secreted from the retina, gastrointestinal tract tissues, skin, platelets, and bone marrow. Melatonin production is described in **Figure 1**.

 IntechOpen

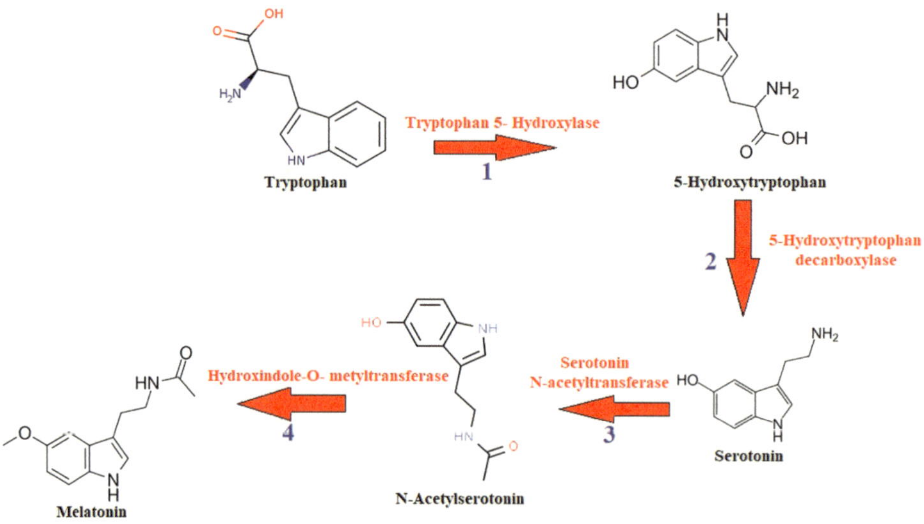

Figure 1.
Synthesis of melatonin from tryptophan.

Melatonin is given to the body by oral or intravenous which is rapidly absorbed and metabolized mainly in the liver and secondarily in the kidneys. Two types of membrane receptors [MT1 and MT2] and one type of cytoplasmic receptor [MT3] for melatonin were determined in humans [5]. Melatonin is both a lipid- and water-soluble hormone, with three types of high-affinity G-protein-coupled receptors mainly MT1, MT2, and MT3. MT1 is a receptor located mainly in the suprachiasmatic nucleus (SCN) and to a lesser extent in the pituitary and cerebral vascular systems (CVSs). MT2 is found in the retina. In addition, melatonin receptors in coronary arteries have been demonstrated [5]. Besides CVSs, melatonin receptors are found in multiple tissues. MT3 receptors are nuclear binding sites of melatonin located in the cytosol [6], acting as an enzyme and responsible for the detoxification of harmful agents. MT1 receptors are mainly found in the cardiovascular system. It can also be found in the immune system, placenta, retina, spleen, liver, breast, kidney, skin, testis, ovary, pancreas, adrenal cortex, retina, and brain [4]. MT2 is found in the immune system, mammary glands, retinal pituitary gland, adipose tissue, SCN, blood vessels, testicles, gastrointestinal tract, kidney, and skin.

2. Melatonin and CVDs relationship

Nowadays, deaths due to CVD are among the most important causes of death, approximately one-third of all deaths. Considering the pathophysiology of cardiovascular diseases, preventive measures and effective substances will reduce the formation and development of these disorders [7].

Melatonin is gaining more and more important in the pathophysiology of CVD. Because low secretion of melatonin has been reported to be associated with various CVDs, including myocardial infarction (MI), coronary heart disease, congestive heart failure, and nocturnal hypertension [8, 9]. Furthermore, working in illuminated environments also causes glucose intolerance, insulin resistance, metabolic circadian irregularity and sleep disturbance with aging, and lack of melatonin secretion [10].

Melatonin receptors have been identified within the cardiovascular system, including various vascular tissues. Hypertension and peripheral vasoconstriction have been reported in animals undergoing pinealectomy [8, 11].

3. Antioxidant and free radical scavenger activity of melatonin

Melatonin is a powerful antioxidant substance and also has protective effects on the mitochondria [12–15]. A study showed beneficial effects on plasma MDA, GSH, PCO, and NO levels after the administration of 5 mg of melatonin (twice a day) for 12 weeks in diabetic patients [15]. Melatonin performs its antioxidant and free radical scavenging activity through two main mechanisms. In the first mechanism, melatonin binds to the MT3 receptor and acts as an antioxidant by suppressing the electron transfer reactions of quinones [16]. In the second pathway, they scavenge free radicals [17]. Depending on the dose of endogenous or exogenous melatonin, it acts by receptor-dependent or receptor-independent mechanisms [18].

Additionally, the aforementioned two mechanisms, melatonin indirectly increases antioxidant enzymes such as glutathione peroxidase, glutathione reductase superoxide dismutase, and glucose-6-phosphate dehydrogenase and suppresses molecular damage under conditions of severe oxidative stress [19]. Antioxidant enzymes realize this stimulation via MT1 and MT2 receptors. Due to its high lipophilicity, melatonin can easily pass through cell membranes and reach intracellular compartments including the nucleus and mitochondria. Melatonin reduces cell death while maintaining normal mitochondrial function [20].

Melatonin and metabolites of melatonin [cyclic 3-hydroxymelatonin and N1-acetyl-N2-formyl-5-methoxyquinuramine] are free radical scavengers [18]. Therefore, melatonin and its metabolites support the main molecule in terms of the antioxidant effect. In addition, the total antioxidant capacity of melatonin is higher than that of other known antioxidants such as vitamin E and vitamin C under in vivo and in vitro conditions [4]. Recent studies have reported that melatonin decreases mammalian Mst1 phosphorylation and increases Sirt3 expression and modulates the autophagic cell death process. Autophagy is a lysosomal cell death process that removes damaged organelles and misfolded proteins to maintain cellular homeostasis [21]. Disruption in autophagy causes cardiac hypertrophy [22], heart failure [Thomas et al. 2013], and ischemia/reperfusion [I/R] damage [23]. Melatonin administration alleviated the left ventricular remodeling. Melatonin also reduces cardiac dysfunction in diabetic animals [24] and has shown a significant protective effect on ischemia/reperfusion [I/R] injury and hypertension [23, 25].

4. Melatonin and immune system

The immunological role of melatonin was first reported by Maestroni et al. in 1987 [26]. In the study, it was observed that immune functions were suppressed in conditions where melatonin formation was inhibited by continuous exposure to light or the administration of β-adrenergic receptor blockers at night. This effect of melatonin is not evident under normal conditions. However, the effect becomes evident in cases where the immune system is suppressed, such as aging, viral diseases, corticosteroid use, or acute stress [27–29]. In another study, they reported that suppression of immune functions as a result of soft tissue trauma and hemorrhagic shock in mice was reversed with melatonin, and that chronic melatonin treatment increased natural killer cell activity in humans [30]. The effects of melatonin against immunosuppression or enhancing immune functions are related to its binding to specific receptors on T-helper lymphocytes. The binding of melatonin to these receptors increases the secretion of gamma-interferon, IL-2, or opioid peptides. In addition, the administration of melatonin in tumor-formed mice protected blood cells from the toxic effects of chemotherapeutic drugs [29]. Also, some studies reported the melatonin anti-inflammatory effect in periodontitis [31–36]. However, melatonin also shows an immunodepressant effect in relation to the dose. At high pharmacological doses (> 100 mg/kg BW), melatonin suppresses antibody formation [29]. The inhibitory effect of melatonin on the immune response and its antioxidant effect suggest that melatonin may be beneficial in organ transplantation. In addition, the lack of toxicity supports that this agent is an agent that can be used safely in transplantation [27].

5. Mechanisms for a relation cardiovascular disease

Melatonin stimulates the phospholipase C pathway by activating MT1 and MT2 receptors via the G inhibitor protein. This results in an increase in Ca^{++} concentration and leads to phosphorylation of protein kinase C (PKC). PKC activates the protein/activation transcription factor cAMP-responsive element-binding protein and activating transcription factor (CREB-ATF). This pathway immediately regulates early gene transcription and thus gene transcription regulation and antioxidant enzyme levels. The production of reactive oxygen species (ROS) stimulates the expression of genes involved in inflammatory processes in the cell. Thus, the transcription of nuclear factor kappa (NF-kB) increases the expression of these inflammatory genes. Inactive NF-kB resides in the cytoplasm due to an inhibitory subunit [I-kB]. I-κB is phosphorylated, and NF-κB is translocated into the nucleus via stimulation of the cells by oxidative stress. PKC may also activate NF-κB, and it binds to the κB response element in its target genes' enhancer and promoter regions. Some of these are located in the promoter regions of the major antioxidant enzymes. Thus, an early cellular response to oxidative stress activates the antioxidant systems [37–39]. The role of melatonin on the protein kinase C (PKC) and activating transcription factor (CREB-ATF) pathway is described in **Figure 2**.

Recent studies have reported the effects of melatonin [receptor-dependent and non-receptor-mediated] on the cardiovascular system. Melatonin causes vasoconstriction in cerebral arteries and vasodilation in peripheral vascular beds. Myocardial infarction (MI) risk, coronary heart patients with sudden death risk, high LDL-cholesterol levels, and also in hypertensive patients, melatonin levels were found to be low [40–42]. The vasodilator effect of melatonin also plays an important role in inducing sleep through thermoregulation. The effects of free radicals play an important role in oxidant damage, especially in the cardiovascular system, caused by high blood pressure [43]. In addition, a decrease was observed in echocardiographic measurements, biochemical parameters in the myocardium, and measured tissue damage parameters in experimental hypertension with melatonin administration [44] (**Figure 2**). It is known that inflammation plays an important role in coronary heart diseases including atherosclerosis. Active compounds released by immune cells that

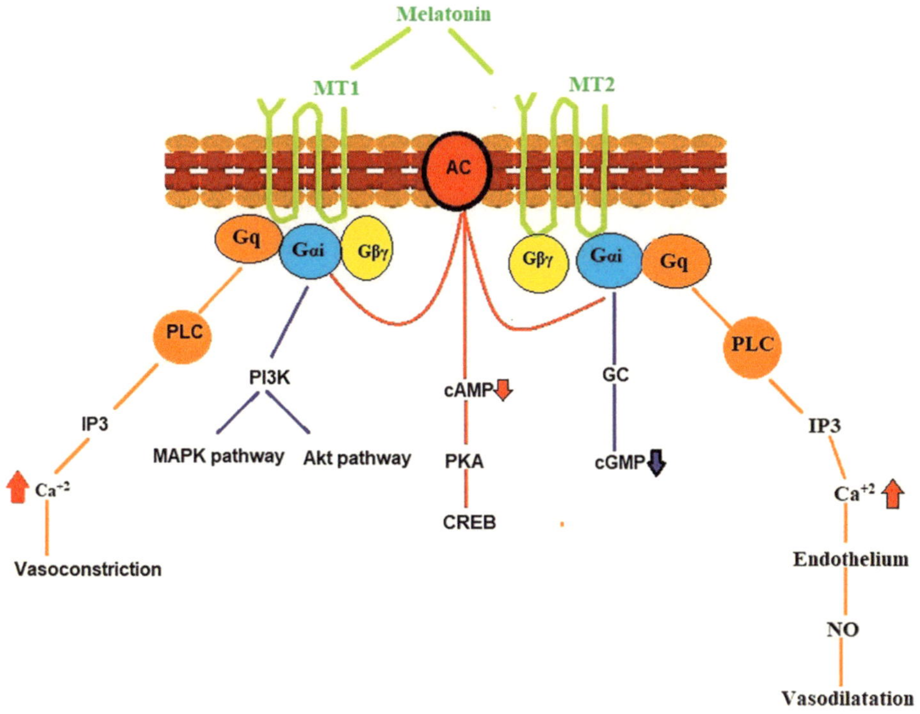

Figure 2.
MT 1 and MT 2 melatonin receptor signaling. PKA, protein kinase a; cAMP response element-binding protein; MT, melatonin receptor; Akt, threonine protein kinase B [PKB; also known as Akt]; cyclic adenosine monophosphate; cGMP, cyclic guanosine monophosphate; CREB, IP3, inositol trisphosphate; MAPK, mitogen-activated protein kinase.

become dominant in the early stages of atherosclerosis cause the progression of both atherosclerotic lesions and inflammation. An increased incidence of MI and sudden death in coronary heart muscles have been associated with decreased melatonin levels in these patients. In animals with hyperlipidemia fed with high cholesterol, melatonin administration was found to be protective of the aorta by increasing antioxidant enzyme activities in these animals [45].

5.1 The relationship between melatonin and blood pressure

It has been reported in previous studies that blood pressure and catecholamine levels are related to circadian rhythm. Blood serum melatonin levels of patients with hypertension were found to be low [46]. In addition, melatonin administration has been found to decrease blood pressure in hypertensive and normotensive patients [47, 48]. Yıldız and Akdemir investigated the endogenous role of melatonin on arterial elasticity and blood pressure for arterial expandability as assessed by aortic pulse wave velocity [49]. Melatonin reduces vascular pressure through its receptor on the arterial wall or by modulation of autonomic activity [50]. It has been reported that the vasodilator effect of melatonin can be achieved by inhibiting the methylation of endothelial nitric oxide synthase [51]. In some studies, melatonin has been reported to cause vasoconstriction by inducing norepinephrine signaling as a result of melatonin binding to MT1 receptors on smooth muscle cells [52].

Doolen et al. demonstrated a vasodilator effect on rat caudal arteries by administering 4-phenyl-2-acetamidotetralin, a selective MT2 agonist [53]. According to our current knowledge, MT1 receptor activation causes vasoconstriction, while MT2 receptor activation causes vasodilation [53]. Differential responses of the vascular bed to melatonin uptake are associated with different distribution of melatonin receptors.

5.2 The relationship between melatonin and lipid profile

Melatonin positively affects the lipid profile regarding CVD [54]. The intestinal system and liver play a significant active role in the metabolism and production of lipoproteins. Lipids are digested in the intestine system and then transported from the intestine to the liver as chylomicrons. In the liver, it is biochemically transformed, and free fatty acids are converted to triglycerides (TGs) and phospholipids. They are transported into the blood system by lipoproteins. LDL is the form of lipoprotein that carries cholesterol into cells, and it also tends to be oxidized by free oxygen radicals, damaging cells and promoting inflammation [55]. Some studies have focused on the damage caused by highly reactive oxygen species (ROS), which leads to atherosclerotic progression. An experimental study reported that melatonin supplementation with an atherogenic diet increased atherosclerotic lesions in the proximal aorta in hypercholesterolemic mice, in contrast to the majority of other studies, by increasing the susceptibility of atherogenic lipoproteins to γ-radiolysis and $Cu2+$ oxidation [55]. In another study, the administration of melatonin for 14 months in individuals with fatty liver disease (not alcoholic) showed that LDL and triglyceride levels decreased compared to the health group [56]. Melatonin administration reduced blood pressure as well as LDL-cholesterol levels [54]. Melatonin protects macromolecules from oxidation damage with its direct effect and free radical scavenging effect by stimulating antioxidant enzymes. The positive effects of melatonin on the lipid profile may be related to its anti-inflammatory and antioxidative effects. In addition, melatonin decreases lipid levels by increasing the conversion of endogenous cholesterol to bile acids and suppresses cholesterol synthesis and accumulation.

6. Recommendations for future research

Although the inflammation hypothesis provides a plausible and compelling explanation for CVDs, including their association with atherosclerosis, more research is needed to define the mechanisms linking the two diseases and how best to manage them to reduce the risk of inflammation and ROS production. Specific questions that the consensus panel believes should be addressed in future research include as follows:

1. Is inflammation an independent risk factor for CVD?

2. If inflammation is an independent risk factor for atherosclerosis and CVD, what is the mechanism of the association, and at what stage[s] of atherogenesis is it important?

3. Regardless of whether inhibition of ROS production is an independent risk factor for atherosclerosis and CVD, should risk factors for CVD in these situations be treated more aggressively than current guidelines recommend for the general population?

DOI: http://dx.doi.org/10.5772/intechopen.106085

Conflict of interest

The authors declare no conflict of interest.

Author details

Hülya Kara[1] and Adem Kara[2]*

1 Faculty of Veterinary Medicine, Department of Anatomy, Atatürk University, Erzurum, Turkey

2 Faculty of Science, Department of Molecular Biology and Genetics, Erzurum Technical University, Erzurum, Turkey

*Address all correspondence to: ademkara36@erzurum@edu.tr

References

[1] Lerner AB, Case JD, Takahashi Y, et al. Isolation of melatonin, the pineal gland factor that lightens melanocytes. Journal of the American Chemical Society. 1958;**80**:2587. DOI: 10.1021/ja01543a060

[2] Altun A, Ugur AB. Melatonin: Therapeutics and clinical utilization. International Journal of Clinical Practice. 2007;**61**:835-845. DOI: 10.1111/j. 1742-1241.2006.01191.x

[3] Pandi-Perumal SR, Bahammam AS, Ojike NI, et al. Melatonin and human cardiovascular disease. Journal of Cardiovascular Pharmacology and Therapeutics. 2017;**22**:122-132. DOI: 10.1177/1074248416660622

[4] Pandi-Perumal SR, Trakht I, Srinivasan V, et al. Physiological effects of melatonin: Role of melatonin receptors and signal transduction pathways. Progress in Neurobiology. 2008;**85**:335-353. DOI: 10.1016/j. pneurobio.2008.04.001

[5] Ekmekcioglu C, Haslmayer P, Philipp C, et al. 24h variation in the expression of the mt, melatonin receptor subtype in coronary heart disease. Chronobiology International. 2001;**18**:973-985. DOI: 10.1081/ CBI-100107972

[6] Hardeland R, Madrid JA, Tand DX, Reiter RJ. Melatonin the circadian multioscillator system and health: The need for detailed analyses of peripheral melatonin signalling. Journal of Pineal Research. 2011;**52**:139-166. DOI: 10.1111/j.1600-079X.2011.00934.x

[7] Mozos I. Links between shift work, cardiovascular risk and disorders. In: He W, Yu L, editors. Shift Work: Impacts, Disorders and Studies. New York: Nova Science Pub Inc; 2017. pp. 23-44

[8] Baker J, Kimpinski K. Role of melatonin in blood pressure regulation: An adjunct anti-hypertensive agent. Clinical and Experimental Pharmacology & Physiology. 2018;**45**:755-766

[9] Mukherjee D, Ghosh AK, Bandyopadhyay A, Basu A, Datta S, Pattari SK, et al. Melatonin protects against isoproterenol-induced alterations in cardiac mitochondrial energymetabolizing enzymes, apoptotic proteins, and assists in complete recovery from myocardial injury in rats. Journal of Pineal Research. 2012;**53**:166-179

[10] Cipolla-Neto J, Amaral FG, Afeche SC, Tan DX, Reiter RJ. Melatonin, energy metabolism, and obesity: A review. Journal of Pineal Research. 2014;**56**:371-381

[11] Zanoboni A, Forni A, Zanoboni-Muciaccia W, Zanussi C. Effect of pinealectomy on arterial blood pressure and food and water intake inthe rat. Journal of Endocrinological Investigation. 1978;**1**:125-130

[12] Kurhaluk N, Bojkova B, Radkowski M, Zaitseva OV, Kyriienko S, Demkow U, et al. Melatonin and metformin diminish oxidativestress in heart tissue in a ratmodel of high fat diet and mammarycarcinogenesis. Advances in Experimental Medicine and Biology. 2018;**1047**:7-19

[13] Gerush IV, Bevzo VV, Ferenchuk YO. The effect of melatonin on lipid peroxide oxidation, oxidative modification of proteins and mitochondria swelling in the skeletal muscle tissue of rats under

alloxan diabetes. Ukrainian Biochemical Journal. 2018;**90**:62-69

[14] Djordjevic B, Cvetkovic T, Stoimenov TJ, Despotovic M, Zivanovic S, Basic J, et al. Oral supplementation with melatonin reduces oxidative damage and concentrations of inducible nitric oxide synthase, VEGF and matrix metalloproteinase 9 in the retina of rats with streptozotocin/nicotinamide induced pre-diabetes. European Journal of Pharmacology. 2018;**833**:290-297

[15] Raygan F, Ostad Mohammadi V, Bahmani F, Reiter RJ, Asemi Z. Melatonin administration lowers biomarkers of oxidative stress and cardio-metabolic risk in type 2 diabetic patients with coronary heart disease: A randomized, double-blind, placebo-controlled trial. Clinical Nutrition. 2019;**38**:191-196

[16] Nosjean O, Ferro M, Coge F, Beauverger P, Henlin JM, Lefoulon F, et al. Identification of the melatonin-binding site MT3 as the quinone reductase 2. The Journal of Biological Chemistry. 2000;**275**:31311-31317

[17] Tan DX, Manchester LC, Esteban-Zubero E, Zhou Z, Reiter RJ. Melatonin as a potent and inducible endogenous antioxidant: Synthesis and metabolism. Molecules. 2015;**20**:18886-18906

[18] Jockers R, Delagrange P, Dubocovich ML, Markus RP, Renault N, Tosini G, et al. Update on melatonin receptors: IUPHAR review 20. British Journal of Pharmacology. 2016;**173**:2702-2725

[19] Reiter RJ, Tan DX. Melatonin: A novel protective agent against oxidative injury of the ischemic/reperfused heart. Cardiovascular Research. 2003;**58**:10-19

[20] Acuna-Castroviejo D, Escames G, Venegas C, Diaz-Casado ME, Lima-Cabello E, Lopez LC, et al. Extrapinealmelatonin:Sources,regulation, and potential functions. Cellular and Molecular Life Sciences. 2014;**71**:2997-3025

[21] Roohbakhsh A, Shamsizadeh A, Hayes AW, Reiter RJ, Karimi G. Melatonin as an endogenous regulator of diseases: The role of autophagy. Pharmacological Research. 2018;**133**:265-276

[22] Zaglia T, Milan G, Ruhs A, Franzoso M, Bertaggia E, Pianca N, et al. Atrogin-1 deficiency promotes cardiomyopathy and premature death via impaired autophagy. Journal of Clinical Investigation. 2014;**124**:2410-2424

[23] Rodella LF, Favero G, Foglio E, Rossini C, Castrezzati S, Lonati C, et al. Vascular endothelial cells and dysfunctions: Role of melatonin. Frontiers in Bioscience (Elite Edition). 2013;**5**:119-129

[24] Zhang M, Lin J, Wang S, Cheng Z, Hu J, Wang T, et al. Melatonin protects against diabetic cardiomyopathy through Mst1/Sirt3 signaling. Journal of Pineal Research. 2017;**63**:e12418

[25] Yu L, Liang H, Lu Z, Zhao G, Zhai M, Yang Y, et al. Membrane receptordependent Notch1/Hes1 activation by melatonin protects against myocardial ischemia-reperfusion injury: in vivo and in vitro studies. Journal of Pineal Research. 2015;**59**:420-433

[26] Maestroni GJ, Conti A, Pierpaoli W. Role of the pineal gland in immunity: II. Melatonin enhances the antibody response via an opiatergic mechanism. Clinical and Experimental Immunology. 1987;**68**(2):384

[27] Reiter RJ, Maestroni JM. Melatonin in relation to the antioxidative defense and immune systems: Possible implications for cell and organ transplantation. Journal of Molecular Medicine. 1999;**77**:36-39

[28] Reiter RJ, Calvo JR, Karbownik M, QI W, Tan DX. Melatonin and its relation to the immune system and inflammation. Annals of the New York Academy of Sciences. 2000;**917**:376-386

[29] Maestroni GJM. The immunoendocrine role of melatonin. Journal of Pineal Research. 1995;**19**:149-165

[30] Wichmann MW, Zelleneger R, DeMaso CM, Ayala A, Chaudry IH. Melatonin administration attenuates depressed immune functions after trauma-hemorrhage. The Journal of Surgical Research. 1996;**63**:256-262

[31] Kara A, Akman S, Ozkanlar S, Tozoglu U, Kalkan Y, Canakci CF, et al. Immune modulatory and antioxidant effects of melatonin in experimental periodontitis in rats. Free Radical Biology and Medicine. 2013;**55**:21-26

[32] Arabacı T, Kermen E, Özkanlar S, Köse O, Kara A, Kızıldağ A, et al. Therapeutic effects of melatonin on alveolar bone resorption after experimental periodontitis in rats: A biochemical and immunohistochemical study. Journal of Periodontology. 2015;**86**(7):874-881

[33] Kose O, Arabaci T, Kara A, Yemenoglu H, Kermen E, Kizildag A, et al. Effects of melatonin on oxidative stress index and alveolar bone loss in diabetic rats with periodontitis. Journal of Periodontology. 2016;**87**(5):e82-e90

[34] Köse O, Arabaci T, Kizildag A, Erdemci B, Özkal Eminoğlu D, Gedikli S, et al. Melatonin prevents radiation-induced oxidative stress and periodontal tissue breakdown in irradiated rats with experimental periodontitis. Journal of Periodontal Research. 2017;**52**(3):438-446

[35] Ozkanlar S, Kara A, Sengul E, Simsek N, Karadeniz A, Kurt N. Melatonin modulates the immune system response and inflammation in diabetic rats experimentally-induced by alloxan. Hormone and Metabolic Research. 2016;**48**(2):137-144

[36] Gedikli S, Gelen V, Sengul E, Ozkanlar S, Gur C, Agırbas O, et al. Therapeutic effects of melatonin on liver and kidney damages in intensive exercise model of rats. Endocrine, Metabolic & Immune Disorders-Drug Targets [Formerly Current Drug Targets-Immune, Endocrine & Metabolic Disorders]. 2015;**15**(4):308-314

[37] Rezzani R, Rodella LF, Bonomini F, Tengattini S, Bianchi R, Reiter RJ. Beneficial effects of melatonin in protecting against cyclosporine A-induced cardiotoxicity are receptor mediated. Journal of Pineal Research. 2006;**41**:288-295

[38] Tomas-Zapico C, Coto-Montes A. A proposed mechanism to explain the stimulatory effect of melatonin on antioxidative enzymes. Journal of Pineal Research. 2005;**39**:99-104

[39] Rodriguez C, Mayo JC, Sainz RM, et al. Regulation of antioxidant enzymes: A significant role for melatonin. Journal of Pineal Research. 2004;**36**:1-9

[40] Dubocovich ML, Markowska M. Functional MT1 and MT2 melatonin receptors in mammals. Endocrine. 2005;**27**:101-110

[41] Paulis L, Simko F. Blood pressure modulation and cardiovascular

protection by melatonin: Potential mechanisms behind. Physiological Research. 2007;**56**:671-684

[42] Sewerynek E. Melatonin and the cardiovascular system. Neuro Endocrinology Letters. 2002;**23**(Suppl 1): 79-83

[43] Campese VM. Oxidative stress and sympathetic activity in hypertension. American Journal of Hypertension. 2010;**23**:456

[44] Erşahin M, Sehirli O, Toklu HZ, Süleymanoglu S, Emekli Alturfan E, Yarat A, et al. Melatonin improves cardiovascular function and ameliorates renal, cardiac and cerebral damage in rats with renovascular hypertension. Journal of Pineal Research. 2009;**47**:97-106

[45] Şener G, Balkan J, Cevikbaş U, Keyer-Uysal M, Uysal M. Melatonin reduces cholesterol accumulation and prooxidant state induced by high cholesterol diet in the plasma, the liver and probably in the aorta of C57BL/6J mice. Journal of Pineal Research. 2004;**36**:212-216

[46] Zeman M, Dulkova K, Bada V, Herikova I. Plasma melatonin concentrations in hypertensive with dipping and non-dipping blood pressure profile. Life Sciences. 2005;**76**:1795-1803. DOI: 10.1016/j.lfs.2004.08.034

[47] Scheer FA, Van Motfrans GA, van Someren EJ, Mairuhu G, Buijs RM. Daily nighttime melatonin reduces blood pressure in male patients with essential hypertension. Hypertension. 2004;**43**:192-197. DOI: 10.1161/01.HYP.0000113293.15186.3b

[48] Borghi C, Cicero AF. Nutraceuticals with clinically detectable blood pressure lowering effect: A review of available randomized clinical trials and their meta-analyses. British Journal of Clinical Pharmacology. 2017;**83**:163-171. DOI: 10.1111/bcp.12902

[49] Yıldız M, Akdemir O. Assessment of the effects of physiological release of melatonin on arterial distensibility and blood pressure. Cardiology in the Young. 2009;**19**:198-203. DOI: 10.1017/S1047951109003692

[50] Arangino S, Cagnacci A, Angiolucci M, et al. Effects of melatonin on vascular reactivity, catecholamine levels, and blood pressure in healthy men. The American Journal of Cardiology. 1999;**83**:1417-1419. DOI: 10.1016/S0002-9149(99)00112-5

[51] Rexhaj E, Pireva A, Paoloni-Giacobino A, et al. Prevention of vascular dysfunction and arterial hypertension in mice generated by assisted reproductive technologies by addition of melatonin to culture media. American Journal of Physiology. Heart and Circulatory Physiology. 2015;**309**:1151-1156. DOI: 10.1152/ajpheart.00621.2014

[52] Vishwanathan M, Laitinen JT, Saavedra JM. Expression of melatonin receptors in arteries involved in thermoregulation. Proceedings of the National Academy of Sciences. 1990;**87**:6200-6203. DOI: 10.1073/pnas.87.16.6200

[53] Doolen S, Krause DN, Dubocovich ML, Duckles SP. Melatonin mediates two distinct responses in vascular smooth muscle. European Journal of Pharmacology. 1998;**345**:67-69. DOI: 10.1016/S0014-2999(98)00064-8

[54] Kozirog M, Poliwczak AR, Duchnowicz P, Koter Michalak M, Joanna S, Bronce M. Melatonin treatment improves blood pressure, lipid profile,

and parameters of oxidative stress in patients with metabolic syndrome. Journal of Pineal Research. 2011;**50**:261-266. DOI: 10.1111/j.1600-079X.2010.00835.x

[55] Tailleux A, Torpier G, Bonnefont-Rousselot D, et al. Daily melatonin supplementation in mice increases atherosclerosis in proximal aorta. Biochemical and Biophysical Research Communications. 2002;**293**:1114-1123. DOI: 10.1016/S0006-291X(02)00336-4

[56] Celinski K, Konturek PC, Slomka M, et al. Effects of treatment with melatonin and tryptophan on liver enzymes, parameters of fat metabolism and plasma levels of cytokines in patients with non-alcoholic fatty liver disease-14 months follow up. Journal of Physiology and Pharmacology. 2014;**65**:75-82

Chapter 6

Melatonin Pretreatment Effect in a Parkinson Disease Experimental Model Induced by the Inhalation of Manganese in Mice

Maria Rosa Avila-Costa, Mariana Stephania Rodríguez-Alcántara, Ana Luisa Gutierréz-Valdez, José Luis Ordoñez-Librado, Vianey Rodríguez-Lara, Leonardo Reynoso-Erazo, Claudia Dorado-Martínez, Cesar Alfonso Garcia Caballero, Enrique Montiel-Flores, Javier Sanchez-Betancourt, Rocío Tron-Alvarez, Patricia Aley-Medina and Jesús Espinosa-Villanueva

Abstract

Parkinson disease (PD) is characterized by dopaminergic neuron loss of the substantia nigra compacta (SNc) and motor alterations. Here, we used the experimental model of inhalation of the mixture of manganese chloride ($MnCl_2$) and manganese acetate Mn $(OAc)_3$ for inducing PD. This model causes bilateral and progressive degeneration of the SNc dopaminergic neurons. Melatonin has antioxidant properties and it has been suggested that it contributes to the protective effect in neurodegenerative diseases. Therefore, we aimed to determine whether melatonin pretreatment protects against the Mn-induced alterations. Before Mn inhalation, three groups were trained for motor performance (1. control group, 2. Mn mixture exposed without pretreatment, and 3. melatonin-pretreated/Mn-exposed groups) for motor tests. The motor coordination was evaluated through the single-pellet reaching task and the beam-walking test. After five months, all the animals were sacrificed. Dendritic spines were counted in the striatum medium-sized spiny neurons and the number of TH-immunoreactive neurons in the SNc. Our findings show that the melatonin-pretreated animals had better motor coordination and less dendritic spines and TH immunoreactive neuron loss than the Mn-inhalation-only group. Therefore, melatonin pretreatment has a neuroprotective effect and could be considered an alternative treatment before the more severe PD symptoms appear.

Keywords: melatonin pretreatment, Parkinson disease, manganese inhalation, motor performance, dendritic spines, TH immunohistochemistry

1. Introduction

Parkinson disease (PD) is the second most prevalent neurodegenerative disease after Alzheimer's [1–3]. This disorder usually occurs in middle/advanced ages with gradual progression and prolonged evolution. It is also disabling and incurable. The estimated prevalence of PD is 0.3% in the general population and 3% in those older than 60. James Parkinson described PD in 1817 where he refers to the "shaking palsy" syndrome as "involuntary trembling movements with decreased muscle strength, in areas that are not in activity and even when helped; propensity to lean the trunk forward and transition from walking to running, while the senses and intellect remain unchanged" [4]. The first PD symptoms are evident after 80% dopamine depletion [5].

PD is a neurodegenerative disorder in which neuronal loss and reactive gliosis are observed in dopamine-synthesizing neurons in the substantia nigra compacta (SNc), along with alpha-synuclein inclusions called Lewy bodies [4]. Biochemical studies show a decrease in dopamine concentration in the striatum, which is why it is considered a disease of the nigrostriatal dopaminergic system [1, 4]. This loss is probably caused by the overexpression and misfolding of proteins such as α-synuclein, which generates structural malformations that lead to mitochondrial respiratory chain dysfunction and Lewy body formation [6, 7].

The dopaminergic neuron degeneration begins some years before PD is symptomatic and makes it difficult to establish the cause of the development of the disease [8]. Some genetic and environmental factors have been related to the etiology of the disease [4, 9]. Although it is known that in 10% of cases, the origin is genetic of Mendelian transmission [9–12], the vast majority (90%) are classified as sporadic PD, defined as polygenic and multifactorial [4, 10]. For this reason, different hypotheses have been established about its origin, some of which include:

- Environmental factors: Various epidemiological studies suggest the relationship between industrialization and the use of agrochemicals as factors in the incidence of PD, such as paraquat and rotenone [9, 13, 14].

- Genetic factors: Recently, several genes related to susceptibility and risk loci associated with PD have been identified. Research has focused on mutations in the SNCA genes (PARK 1/PARK 4), which is the first dominant autonomic transmission gene identified in PD [12], and the mutation in the GBA gene, which is the most significant genetic risk factor for developing PD [15]. The LRRK2 gene (PARK 8) is the most frequent form, representing 4% of hereditary PD [16]. Three genes are associated with PD and involved in Lewy body formation: PARK 1, PARK 2, and PARK [17].

- Oxidative stress: The oxygen oxidative properties play an essential role in biological phenomena and can cause damage within cells, mainly through the formation of reactive oxygen species (ROS) such as hydrogen peroxide (H_2O_2), hydroxyl radicals ($OH^•$), and superoxide (O_2^-) [18]. In PD, it has been reported that oxidative stress is the leading cause of SNc dopaminergic neurons deterioration [19]; neuronal death in the SNc can be caused by: (a) increased DA turnover resulting in excess H_2O_2 formation; (b) glutathione peroxidase deficiency, which consequently decreases the ability to clean H_2O_2, and (c) increase in reactive iron, which promotes the $OH^•$ formation. In PD, the SNc cells appear to be in a high oxidative stress state, which is assumed by the increase in lipid, protein, and DNA oxidation products; in the SNc of parkinsonian patients, it is possible to detect oxidative alterations using different markers such as malondialdehyde, which is up to 10 times higher than its average value [19].

- Mitochondrial dysfunction: Currently, it has been proposed that the mechanism of action of a large number of the toxic agents used as PD models involves the inhibition of mitochondrial complexes I and IV and ROS generation so that the role of the mitochondria during the development of PD is fundamental [20–22]. The first evidence was reported in MPTP-induced Parkinson's that produces complex I deficiency and oxidative damage only in the SNc, conferring toxicity and neuronal death [23].

1.1 Parkinson disease experimental models

Although PD etiology is still not fully understood, animal models have provided essential information. Based on clinical and experimental discoveries, PD was the first neurodegenerative disease to be modeled and, later, to be treated by neurotransmitter replacement therapy [13]. The typical PD models (**Table 1**) are designed to induce nigrostriatal dopaminergic neuronal loss, commonly with 6-hydroxydopamine (6-OHDA), 1-methyl-4-phenyl-1,2,3,6-tetrahydropyridine (MPTP), paraquat, or rotenone [11, 13, 14, 24].

Most of these models induce mitochondrial dysfunction and produce ROS, but none of them completely replicates PD pathology and symptoms observed in humans [11]. MPTP and 6-OHDA are neurotoxins that promptly and selectively destroy dopaminergic neurons (1–3 days), whereas PD pathogenesis gradually develops throughout decades [13, 25].

Recently, we developed a novel PD experimental model in mice [26, 27] and rats [28] by the inhalation of the mixture of two manganese (Mn) compounds, manganese chloride ($MnCl_2$) and manganese acetate ($Mn(OAc)_3$). After 5 months (mice) or 6 months (rats) of Mn mixture inhalation, the animals presented a significant loss of SNc tyrosine hydroxylase-positive (TH^+) neurons; the loss of these neurons was 67.58% [27] and 71% [28]. Further on, we confirmed that the alterations were of dopaminergic origin since the motor alterations improved at the level of the controls with Levodopa (L-DOPA) treatment [28, 29]. In short, after 5 or 6 months

Model	Characteristics	Disadvantages
6-OHDA[a]	The first established model. The neuronal degeneration is in 24 h. Enters via dopamine transporter (DAT) and inhibits the mitochondrial respiratory chain.	Unilateral injection, acute model. Unilateral damage, measurable by ipsi or contralateral rotations.
MPTP[b]	Humans and monkeys have the same symptoms/histopathology and response to L-DOPA. It is transformed to MPP+ in the glia and enters through the DAT	Lower susceptibility in rodents, the administration is acute or subacute. In rodents, there is recovery.
Rotenone	Damage to the SNc and cytoplasmic inclusions, similar to Lewi bodies. Inhibition of mitochondrial respiratory chain.	Neuronal selectivity, not all animals are affected.

[a]6-hydroxydopamine.
[b]1-methyl-4-phenyl-1,2,3,6-tetrahydropyridine.

Table 1.
Some PD experimental models.

of Mn mixture inhalation, striatal dopamine was reduced by 71%, and SNc showed a significant decrease in the number of TH^+ neurons. The animals developed akinesia, postural instability, and tremor, providing evidence that $MnCl_2/Mn(OAc)_3$ mixture inhalation produces comparable morphological, neurochemical, and behavioral alterations to those observed in PD, suggesting a useful experimental model for the study of this neurodegenerative disease. Additionally, Mn inhalation is progressive and bilateral, making it more reliable.

1.2 Parkinson disease treatments

Current treatments include pharmacological and surgical approaches, but despite advances, none of these manages to modify the clinical course of the disease [30]. The most common therapeutic approaches are mentioned below:

1.2.1 Cell therapy and neurotrophic factors

The main objective of this treatment is to replace the altered cells with others that can replace their function. Usually, these neurons implanted in the SNc are dopamine-producing cells, and, ideally, they restore the functional connectivity of the nigrostriatal pathway [31, 32]. However, the most frequent drawbacks of cell therapy are infections or rejections [33].

Neurotrophic factors also regulate the proliferation, survival, migration, and differentiation of all cell types of the nervous system; in addition to regulating the establishment of adequate connections, both in embryonic and adult development phases, including the glial cell-derived neurotrophic factor (GDNF), which is the most appropriate for PD treatment, since it is the most powerful neurotrophic factor described to date [34] exerting a powerful trophic action on dopaminergic neurons [35].

1.2.2 Dopaminergic agonists

Bromocriptine was the first proposed dopaminergic agonist. It is used for the initial stages of PD because it delays the motor complications induced by long-term L-DOPA administration [36, 37]. Avila-Costa et al. [38] reported that the treatment with bromocriptine in the 6-OHDA-induced PD model attenuated the neurotoxic effect. However, it induces side effects such as nausea, vomiting, confusion, and hallucinations [39, 40]. Apomorphine is another dopaminergic agonist, which can be administered subcutaneously, sublingually, and rectally, but intermittent administration of apomorphine has been reported to cause adverse problems such as skin inflammation, crusting, and nasal obstruction [40, 41].

Another commonly used dopaminergic agonist is pramipexole, which stimulates D3 receptors and, to a lesser extent, D2 and D4 receptors [42], which has been evaluated against placebo, with the demonstration of absolute efficacy in symptom control [43]. Compared to L-DOPA, pramipexole has a lower incidence of dyskinesias and motor fluctuations; however, undesirable effects have been described with this drug, such as alterations in short-term verbal memory, executive functions, and verbal fluency in comparison with patients treated with L-DOPA [44].

The most common PD treatment is with the dopamine precursor L-DOPA. The precursor is used due to the inability of DA to cross the blood–brain barrier [45, 46]; however, L-DOPA loses its efficacy after a few years because neuronal death continues, and therefore the dosage has to be increased, and in most patients, chronic administration of L-DOPA causes dyskinesias [30, 47, 48], which affect the patients to the degree of incapacitating them to continue with their activities [49].

1.2.3 Antioxidants

The proposal to use therapeutic strategies based on drugs with antioxidant properties is because antioxidant enzymes play a significant role in protecting against oxidative stress, which plays a substantial role in PD neurodegeneration [22, 23, 50], some of these, such as vitamin E, coenzyme Q, and melatonin, have been widely proposed as therapeutic strategies [22, 51–54], but they usually are used in combination with some dopaminergic agonists [55].

1.2.4 Melatonin

Melatonin (N-acetyl-5-methoxytryptamine) is a neurohormone, synthesized mainly in the pineal gland from the amino acid tryptophan, which is converted to 5-hydroxytryptamine by the enzymes tryptophan hydrolase and 5-hydroxytryptophan decarboxylase [56]. From this moment on, 5-hydroxytryptamine is transformed into N-acetylserotonin by the action of N-acetyl transferase, the rate-limiting enzyme in melatonin synthesis. Finally, N-acetylserotonin is converted into melatonin by O-methylation through hydroxy indole-O-methyltransferase [57]. Melatonin is involved in multiple biological processes; it mainly regulates circadian rhythms due to its effect on the hypothalamus and the suprachiasmatic nucleus during the dark phase of the photoperiod. However, their functions are much broader in terms of the sites of biosynthesis and action [56, 58]. This molecule has been extensively studied since important antioxidant properties have been attributed to it [59, 60]. It has been reported that it is twice more efficient than vitamin E and four times more efficient than glutathione peroxidase and ascorbic acid [61]. Melatonin acts through two G protein-coupled membrane receptors: MT1 and MT2 [62]. Melatonin also shows an affinity for another binding site, MT3 receptors, which represent a quinone enzyme reductase 2, which may participate in antioxidant protection by removing prooxidant quinones [63].

In 2012, Gutiérrez-Valdez et al. [55] compared the effect of the chronic administration of L-DOPA and melatonin in unilaterally 6-OHDA-lesioned rats where they found that melatonin treatment is capable of protecting the alterations produced by the lesion, suggesting that melatonin may be a possible candidate for the treatment of PD.

As mentioned above, PD is the second most prevalent neurodegenerative disease worldwide, and unfortunately, with the standard treatments, unfavorable side effects have been described that can become very frequent and hinder the patient more. One of the most accepted hypotheses regarding PD etiology is that dopaminergic cell damage is caused by oxidative stress. Therapeutic alternatives have been sought to reduce the secondary damage caused by the treatments, and it has been found that melatonin has important antioxidant properties that could prevent cytological damage and not cause adverse effects, improving the patient's quality of life. Thus, this work investigates the possible protective effect (avoiding or delaying neuronal damage) of melatonin pretreatment through the Mn mixture inhalation as a PD experimental model.

2. Methods

Male CD1 mice (n = 15) with an initial weight of 33 ± 3 g were used; the mice were maintained in 12:12 light/dark cycles, with free access to water and food (except on the days of motor test evaluation). Mice were divided into three groups (see **Table 2**).

2.1 Melatonin pretreatment

The pretreated group was administered, melatonin 10 mg/kg mixed with Nestlé® Cerelac in 0.3 ml water orally in the afternoon (2:30 p.m.); the animals received the dose for 30 days before the $MnCl_2/Mn(OAc)_3$ inhalation.

2.2 Motor evaluation

On day 23 of melatonin administration, the animals of the three groups were trained in the beam walking test and the reaching task.

2.2.1 Beam walking test

This test evaluates the mice's ability to cross a narrow beam (3 mm wide) to reach an enclosed safety platform [64]. A wooden device with two pedestals was used, to which a 1 m long wooden beam with a 15° inclination and 3 mm width was attached (**Figure 1**), where the animals had to walk from the bottom of the device until they reached their home box. During training, animals were placed at the beam start with no inclination and trained over 4r days (four trials per day). Once the animals crossed the beam in a ~20 s interval, they received two more consecutive trials with the inclined beam. The time it took for the animals to cross the beam (total time) [27] was recorded with a stopwatch; a maximum time of 16 s was expected, and if at the end of this time the mouse did not cross, the activity was terminated. The parameters evaluated by this test are motor impairment in slowness, balance, and muscle stiffness, in addition to the alternate use of the limbs [28].

2.2.2 Single pellet reaching task

Besides the beam-walking training, the mice were taught the single pellet reaching task. Each mouse was placed inside an acrylic box 19.5 cm long, 8 cm wide, and 20 cm high, with a 1-cm wide vertical slit in the front of the box. A 0.2 cm thick plastic shelf (8.3 cm long and 3.8 cm wide) through which the animal had to reach a pellet with its preferred forelimb and eat it (**Figure 2**). A total of 20-milligram food pellets were

Group	Inhalation	Treatment
Control n = 5	Deionized water	—
Mn-exposed (n = 5)	$MnCl_2/Mn(OAc)_3$	—
Melatonin pretreated (n = 5)	$MnCl_2/Mn(OAc)_3$	Melatonin (10 mg/kg 30 days before Mn inhalation)

Table 2.
Group distribution.

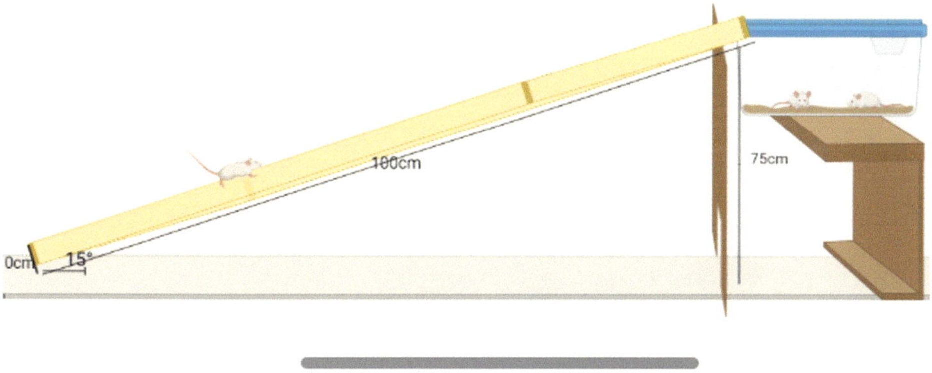

Figure 1.
The beam walking test dimensions. The home box is located at one end of the beam.

placed in indentation spaced 1 cm away from the slit and centered on its edges. Before training and testing, the mice were food-deprived for 24 h. Afterward, they received a restricted diet of ~10 g/kg body weight-adjusted to keep their weight constant. Each animal reached 20 pellets each day during the testing period. Every time the animal took the pellet and brought it to its mouth, it was scored as a success, and when it could not hold it or fell off, the reach was scored as a miss [65]; each animal was given 20 opportunities. The qualitative evaluation comprised the "reaching performance" analysis, the postural shift, impairments in limb extension, aim, supination-pronation of the paw during grasping, and the pellet release into the mouth. The following sequence of movements of the forelimbs was considered [27]: 1. The mouse is placed facing the box slit; 2. Raises the forelimb adjusting its posture to project the limb toward the food pellet, and 3. Holds the pellet, returns its forelimb to the mouth, and introduces it.

This test helps determine the motor deterioration in terms of slowness in the sequence of movements, tremors, and a decrease in strength and precision [28]. The evaluations of both tests were carried out once a week for 5 months.

The inclusion/exclusion criteria of the mice trained to continue with the experiment were those animals that took less than 17 s to perform the test in the case of the beam test. Only those mice that obtained 16 or more successful executions were used for the single pellet reaching task.

2.3 Manganese inhalation

Mn inhalation was performed as described previously by our group [66]. Ten mice were placed in an acrylic compartment inhaling the mixture of 0.04 M $MnCl_2$ and 0.02 M $Mn(OAc)_3$ (Sigma Aldrich Co., Mexico), 1 h twice a week for 5 months. Five control mice inhaled deionized water for the same time. Inhalations were performed in closed acrylic boxes (35 cm wide × 44 cm long and 20 cm high) connected to an ultra-nebulizer (Ultra Neb DeVilbiss, IL, USA) with 10 l/min continuous flux. The ultra-nebulizer produces drops in a 0.5–5 μ range. A vapor trap was placed on the opposing side with a sodium bicarbonate solution to precipitate the residual Mn. During inhalation, mice were constantly monitored for respiration rate, depth, and regularity. The exposure system's temperature, oxygen level, and Mn concentration were continuously examined.

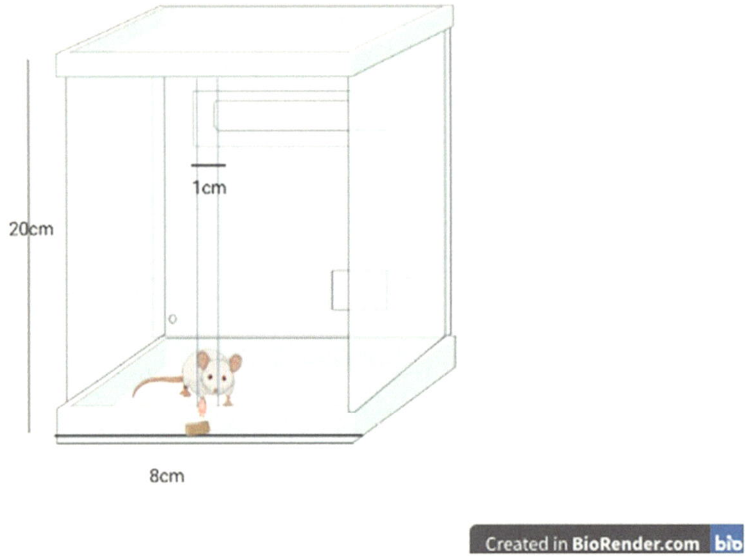

Figure 2.
The single pellet reaching apparatus. The figure shows the dimensions of the reaching box.

After 40 inhalations, when significant motor alterations were observed, mice were anesthetized and sacrificed using a lethal dose of sodium pentobarbital. The animals were perfused via aorta with phosphate buffer saline (0.1 M pH 7.4) containing 2% glutaraldehyde and 2% paraformaldehyde. The brain was removed and placed in a fixative solution for 2 h and processed for tyrosine hydroxylase (TH) immunocytochemistry and Golgi impregnation method.

2.4 Golgi method

Blocks from the striatum were processed for the rapid Golgi method and cut into 90 μm-thick sections [67]. The histological analysis consisted in counting the number of dendritic spines in a 10 μm-long area from five secondary dendrites to 10 medium-sized spiny neurons (MSN) per group on both hemispheres [66].

2.5 TH immunocytochemistry

For immunocytochemistry, coronal sections (50 μm) were obtained on a vibrating microtome through the mesencephalon. Tyrosine hydroxylase (Chemicon International, Inc. CA, USA, 1:1000) immunostaining with the ABC detection method (Vector Lab MI, USA) was performed for light microscope analysis. The analysis was conducted with a computer-assisted system (Image-Pro Plus, Media Cybernetics, L. P. del Mar, CA, USA) connected by a CCD camera to Optiphot 2 microscope (Nikon, Japan). The number of TH^{+}- positive neurons was counted in 1500 μm^2 from seven SNc sections of each mouse [66].

2.6 Statistical analysis

Two-way ANOVA was used to analyze behavioral and cellular data. Group differences were considered statistically significant at $P < 0.05$. When appropriate, *posthoc* comparisons were made with the Tukey test. All analyses were conducted with GraphPad Prism 9 Software for Mac.

3. Results

After 5 months of Mn inhalation, neither clinical alterations nor significant weight changes were detected in the exposed animals compared with controls.

The motor impairment induced by inhaling $MnCl_2/Mn(OAc)_3$ mixture was bilateral and progressive. Melatonin pretreatment showed significant results regarding protection against motor alterations and neuronal degeneration.

3.1 Motor behavior

When evaluating the motor deficit that appeared in the beam-walking test and the single pellet reaching task after 5 months, we observed that the melatonin-pretreated/Mn-exposed group obtained better coordination performance in both cases while the exposed group progressively decreased their motor skills (**Figures 3** and **4**). **Figure 3** depicts the beam-walking test results. The average time taken to cross it was determined; after 14 inhalations, the mice in the Mn mixture-exposed group showed an increase in the time to perform the test, and the melatonin-pretreated/Mn-exposed and control groups remained constant. We found significant differences between melatonin-pretreated/Mn-exposed and Mn-exposed/no treatment groups since the latter had greater difficulty crossing the beam.

Regarding the single pellet reaching task, in **Figure 4** we can observe that during the 5 months, the control group maintained an average of 16 correct answers, while in the Mn-exposed/no treatment group, after the fourth inhalation, the number of successes decreased and dropped to an average of 5; however, the melatonin-pretreated/Mn-exposed group had significant differences compared to the Mn-exposed/no treatment group; it was clear that the motor coordination on melatonin-pretreated mice was not so affected.

Motor qualitative assessment after Mn mixture inhalation/no treatment resulted in tremor and bradykinesia, postural shifts and limb extension impairments (resulting in evident shortened reaches), paw aim, and supination-pronation during grasping and pellet release into the snout (**Figure 5** sequence **B**). Mn-exposed/no treatment mice exhibited abnormal movements when recollecting the pellet after Mn-exposure. The paw is often fully pronated and moves either, laterally over the pellet, or the mouse slaps at the pellet from above. These mice repeatedly could not accurately close their fingers around the pellet and took it to the slot without lifting the paw. Mice also failed to supinate the paw entirely and placed their snout into the slot to retrieve the pellet with the tongue. When the paw was pulled out through the slot, Mn-exposed mice frequently twisted their bodies and "chased" the pellet with the mouth instead of opening the fingers and placing it into the snout. However, when observing the control and the melatonin-pretreated/Mn-exposed groups, those animals advanced their forelimb through the slot and extended their fingers, supinated their paw to present the food to the mouth, and extended their digits to release the food into the snout (see **Figure 5** sequences **A, C**).

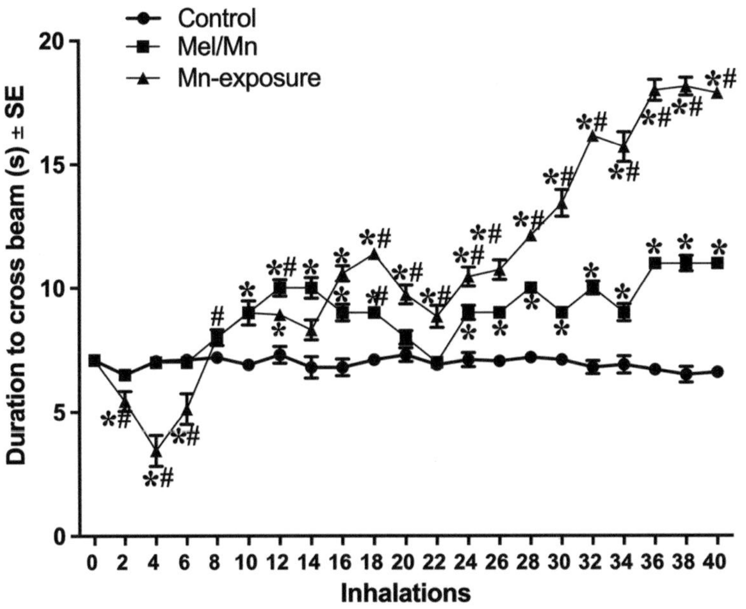

Figure 3.
Mean of the time traveled on the beam ± SE (Mn-exposed groups vs. control group, P < 0.05; # = melatonin-pretreatment vs. Mn-no treatment exposed group; two-way ANOVA followed by Tukey's posthoc test).*

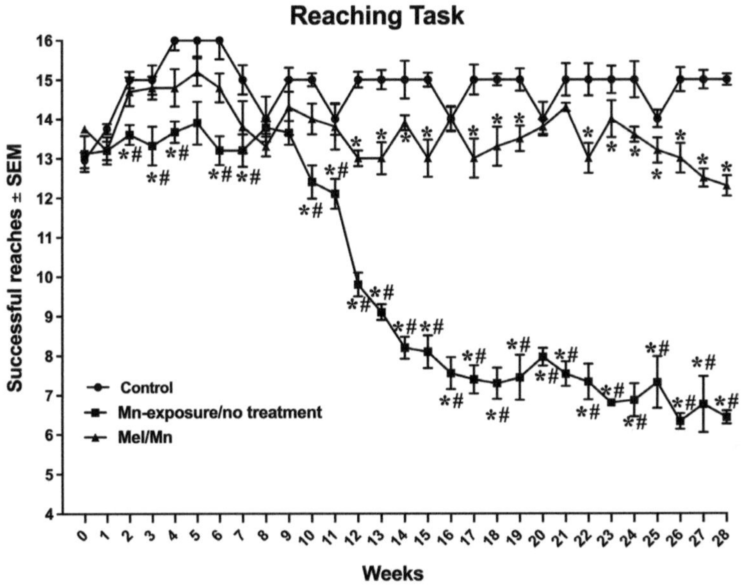

Figure 4.
Reaching success (number of pellets obtained out of 20; mean ± S.E.) by control, melatonin-pretreated/Mn-exposed, and Mn-exposed/no treatment mice in the single-pellet reaching task. Note that the Mn-exposed/no treatment group is impaired after four inhalations (P < 0.001 vs. control group; # P < 0.001 between melatonin-pretreated/Mn-exposed and Mn-exposed/no treatment groups. ANOVA with post hoc test).*

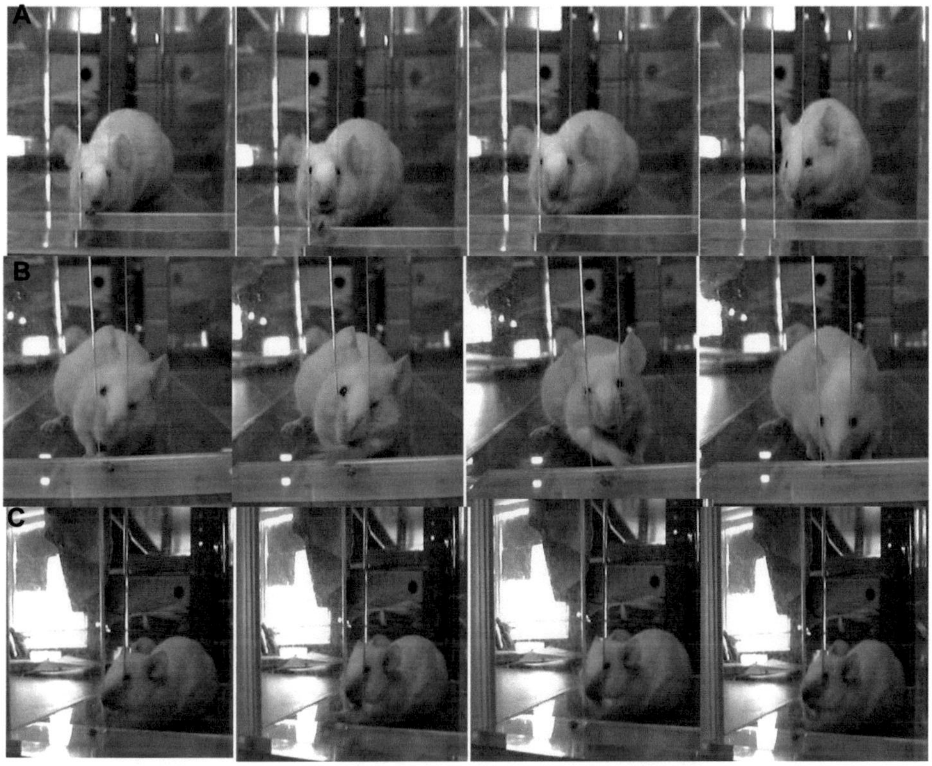

Figure 5.
Representative still frames of the three groups. The control (sequence A) and the melatonin-pretreated/Mn-exposed (sequence C) animals advanced their forelimb through the slot and extended their digits, and also supinated their paw to present the food to the mouth and extended their fingers to release the food into the mouth. In contrast, the Mn mixture-exposed/no treatment mice (sequence B) showed impairments using extreme postural adjustments advancing the limb diagonally through the slot, making many short attempts rather than aligning the limb with the midline of the body. The fingers are concurrently adducted. The paw comes in from the side or slaps laterally, and digits do not contact the food pellet.

3.2 Dendritic spines

When analyzing the number of dendritic spines of the striatal MSN with the Golgi impregnation technique, it was observed (**Figures 6** and **7**) that the number of dendritic spines significantly decreased in the Mn-exposed/no treatment group and in the melatonin-pretreated/Mn-exposed group compared to control; however, it is also shown that the melatonin-pretreated/Mn-exposed group is statistically different from the Mn-only exposed group, in other words, despite having a significant loss of dendritic spines, they lost fewer spines than the group that did not receive treatment.

3.3 TH^+ immunocytochemistry

Regarding the number of SNc dopaminergic neurons (TH^+) (**Figures 8** and **9**), it was observed that the Mn-mixture-exposed/no treatment group presented a significant loss of neurons compared to the melatonin-pretreated/Mn exposed group; both groups had significant differences compared to the control group.

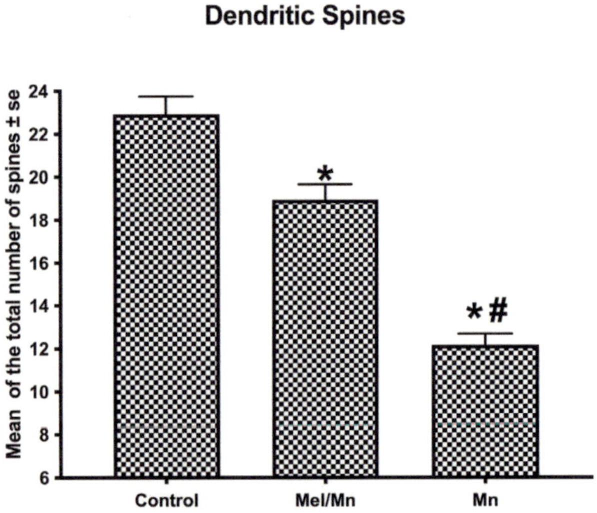

Figure 6.
Golgi-stain analysis. Striatal MSN dendritic spines density of the control, melatonin-pretreated/Mn-exposed, and Mn-no treatment groups (= versus control group, $P < 0.05$; # = melatonin-pretreatment vs. Mn-no treatment exposed group; two-way ANOVA followed by Tukey's posthoc test).*

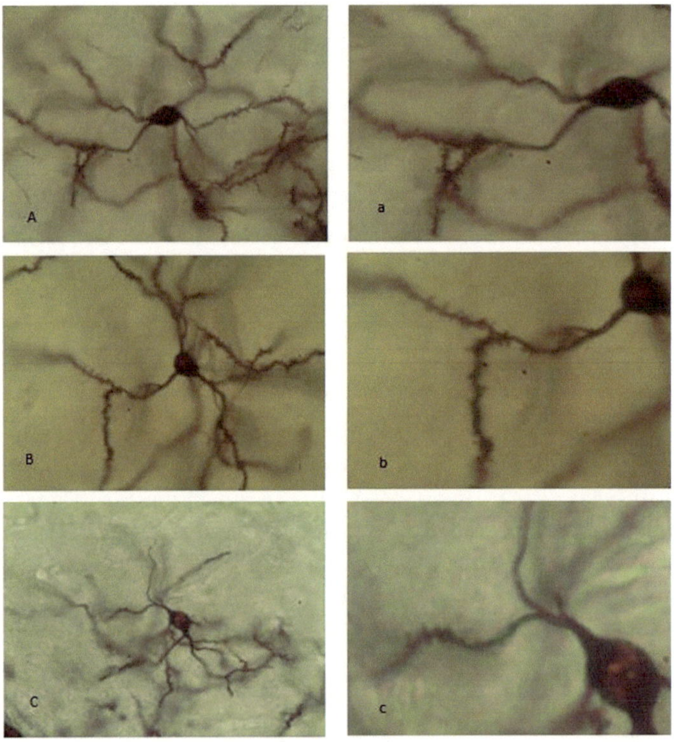

Figure 7.
Dendritic spine density. Photomicrographs of representative Golgi-stained MSN of the striatum from control (A, a), melatonin-pretreated/Mn-exposed (B, b), and Mn mixture-exposed/no treatment groups (C, c). Both Mn-exposed groups had a significant decrease in the total number of spines. However, melatonin-pretreated/ Mn-exposed group showed less dendritic spine loss and an almost a well-preserved dendritic spines density (magnifications: A, B, C 10×; a, b, c 100×).

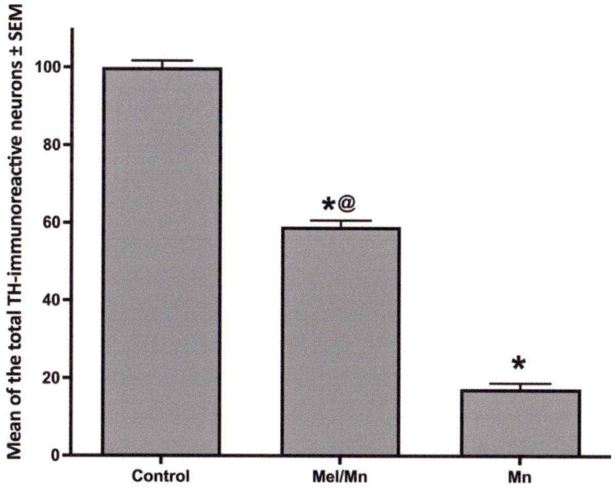

Figure 8.
SNc TH^+ cell count. The data are presented as mean ± SEM. It is observed that both Mn-exposed groups showed a drastic decrease in cells. It is important to note that animals receiving melatonin pretreatment before Mn inhalation lose fewer neurons than Mn-exposed/no treatment group. (= $P < 0.05$ versus control group; # = $P < 0.05$ melatonin-pretreated/Mn exposed group vs. Mn-exposed/no treatment group, ANOVA test followed by Tukey's posthoc test).*

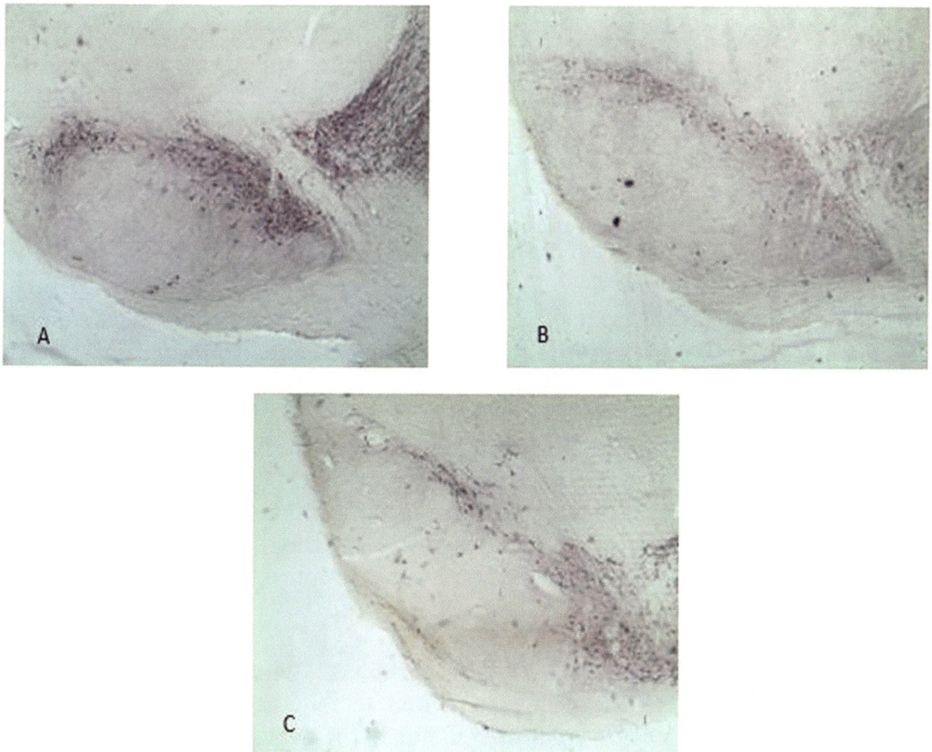

Figure 9.
Representative TH-immunostained from coronal sections containing the SNc of A. Control group; B. Melatonin-pretreated/Mn exposed group, and C. Mn-exposed/no treatment group. Note the great cell loss in the Mn-exposed/no treatment group; although there was a neuronal loss in the pretreated group, it was less drastic than in the untreated-Mn exposed group (magnification 10×).

However, it is observed that, although the melatonin-pretreated/Mn exposed group had a significant loss of TH+ neurons, this loss was less than the group that only inhaled Mn, with significant differences between the two groups.

4. Discussion

PD is a degenerative disorder, determined clinically from movement alterations, and it is reported that the motor symptoms appear relatively late when 80–90% of SNc dopaminergic neurons have been lost [4, 5, 9, 68]. Progressive cell loss leads to increased physical disability, followed by a cognitive decline [1]. Ordoñez-Librado and collaborators [27] indicate that the $MnCl_2/Mn(OAc)_3$ inhalation model is an alternative that allows us to carry out evaluations in the different stages of evolution of the disease since it produces progressive and bilateral degeneration of the SNc dopaminergic neurons in exposed mice, as well as motor alterations, for which it is the model most closely related to what happens in humans [28].

4.1 Motor behavior

Our results showed that in both motor tests, the mice pretreated with melatonin did not have such a drastic decrease in motor coordination as observed in the animals exposed to Mn with no treatment. In previous works from our group, Sánchez-Betancourt et al. [28] and Ordoñez-Librado et al. [26] reported that animals exposed to the mixture of Mn compounds present motor alterations as the number of inhalations increases. Motor alterations are closely related to basal ganglia, which have a fundamental role in the initiation and execution of continuous movement; in other words, they participate in the planning of complex movements [69], for example, in the automatic control of movements such as gait primarily through its interaction with cortical motor areas. However, disruption of this system can lead to gait disturbances as in PD [70]; gait disturbances are common symptoms of parkinsonism [71, 72]; PD patients have a shortened stride length with a shuffling step and reduced speed (festinant) [73]. Our results also agreed with Fernagut et al. [74], who observed that MPTP-lesioned mice presented alterations in the extremities' coordination. In the beam walking test results, the mice exposed to Mn/no treatment did not coordinate their limbs correctly and had great difficulty climbing the beam. This group also manifested akinesia. It is well known that akinesia rapidly becomes intolerable when PD patients are not LD-treated [30]. This symptom was not present in the melatonin-pretreated/Mn exposed animals. According to this, melatonin bioavailability in the brain is observed from the first 30 min after oral administration. It continues to exert its antioxidant properties through its metabolites for extended periods [75, 76], thus facilitating the reduction of abnormal motor behavior.

On the other hand, in the single pellet reaching task, which consists of a series of motor subcomponents [77], since reaching movements are shortened and limb pronation and supination are impaired due to the decrease in dopamine [78] in Mn-exposed mice [27], in humans, we can observe that manual dexterity worsens as PD progresses [79]; Farr and Whishaw [65] mention that rodents reaching movements are very similar to those of humans and, due to this, homology between them is suggested. Whishaw et al. [78] indicated that using this test is helpful in studies of PD subjects to assess movement efficacy and evaluate dopamine denervation. Conversely, regarding the melatonin-pretreated/Mn exposed group, we observed less deterioration even though they inhaled the mixture of Mn compounds. The motor behavior of these animals was very similar to those of the control group. It has been reported that melatonin systemic administration protects SNc dopaminergic neurons against 6-OHDA neurotoxicity in the rat [52, 80]. The effect is accompanied by a significant motor behavior recovery. In this regard, Singh et al. [52] have reported that melatonin pretreated animals and subsequently 6-OHDA-lesioned and treated with melatonin for seven more days showed a diminution in the number of apomorphine-induced rotations, improved posture, and slowness of movement compared to 6-OHDA-lesioned treated with vehicle solution group.

It has also been reported that elevated ROS participate in Mn-neurotoxicity [81–84]; this has been evidenced by the reduction in brain GSH levels and the loss of SOD activity [83]. Melatonin stimulates antioxidant enzymes such as superoxide dismutase (SOD), glutathione peroxidase (GPX), and glutathione reductase (GRd) [76, 85]. These results demonstrate that melatonin might have beneficial effects on PD treatment.

4.2 Dendritic spines

We found a significant dendritic spine loss in both Mn-exposed groups, being more drastic in the Mn-exposed/no treatment group. Our findings agreed with what was reported previously by our group [26, 28]. We found a decrease in the density of dendritic spines after Mn mixture exposure. Also, it has been reported that striatal MSN of *postmortem* PD brains and the brains of PD animal models in rodents and primates show severe spine loss [86–88]. In this regard, Archibald and Tyree [89] suggested that Mn interacts with dopaminergic catechol groups causing dopamine depletion and damage to these neurons; such loss of striatal dopamine is therefore associated with the reduction of MSN dendritic spines as a compensatory mechanism [90] since by reducing the number of dendritic spines, it also decreases the possibility of glutamatergic synaptic contacts [91–93], avoiding death due to excitotoxicity [92, 93] because cortex excitatory innervation [94].

However, we observed that melatonin pretreatment has a protective effect on the nigrostriatal dopaminergic pathway since, as mentioned, the pretreated animals showed better stability and coordination in the motor tests. We can also observe that in the group pretreated with melatonin, the mice had a significant loss of dendritic spines compared to the exposed group. This agrees with what was reported by Anaya-Martinez et al. [80], where they showed that the animals treated with melatonin that were lesioned with 6-OHDA showed improvement at 28 days after the lesion, as well as the administration of melatonin prevented the loss of MSN dendritic spines, suggesting that melatonin can activate some signaling pathways to increase the defense against ROS. Melatonin stimulates the system of antioxidant enzymes [76], such as SOD, GPx, GRd, and catalase [95], preventing lipid peroxidation in the striatum, and preserving a greater number of dopaminergic neurons in the SNc; this can be explained by the free radical scavenging effect of melatonin and some of its metabolites [76]. Therefore, it is likely that due to these properties, melatonin prevents dopaminergic neurons from degenerating, which is evidenced by the preservation of dendritic spines, since by avoiding the loss of TH^+ neurons, dopaminergic transmission to the striatum is maintained, as well as the dendritic spines integrity [96].

4.3 TH+ immunocytochemistry

We observed an intense decrease of TH^+ cells after Mn inhalation in both exposed groups. Our results coincide with Damier et al. [97], who found that PD patients displayed a dopaminergic neurons decrease of up to 95% depending on the time of clinical evolution. Likewise, it has been demonstrated that the medial forebrain bundle unilateral 6-OHDA lesion reduces 98% of the SNc ipsilateral number of TH- immunoreactive neurons [98, 99]. Some studies have found that Mn exposure causes a decrease in the number of SNc dopaminergic neurons since the Mn enters them through the dopamine transporter (DAT) [27, 28, 100, 101], and intracellularly Mn accumulates in the mitochondria via the Ca^{2+} uniport channel [102], inhibiting respiratory chain complex I and thus, promoting the ROS formation [83], leading neurons to oxidative stress and therefore dead. It is known that melatonin increases complex I and IV mitochondrial activity by raising mitochondrial DNA expression [103]. In addition, melatonin's free radical scavenger property neutralizes radicals such as $OH^{\bullet}$ and $O_2^{\bullet -}$ [58]. Our findings showed that melatonin pretreatment partially prevents SNc dopaminergic cell death produced by Mn mixture inhalation. Among the Mn-inhalation consequences are ROS production [81–83] and the complexes I and IV inhibiting the mitochondria electron transport chain [104]. Inhibition of these complexes has also been described in PD patients SNc. This inhibition triggers energy depletion and increases mitochondria free radical concentration [105].

In the present work, for melatonin pretreated/Mn-exposed group, although the TH^+ cell percentage decreases (compared to the control group), the loss was less severe than that observed in the Mn-exposed/no treated group. Melatonin antioxidant effects and its protective characteristic against the uncoupling of the electron transport chain of several toxins in the mitochondria are summarized by Acuña-Castroviejo et al. [106]. These data give rise to further analyses based on this hypothesis. *In vivo* melatonin pretreatment studies in experimental PD models are scarce. These authors also reported that melatonin prevented lipid peroxidation increase and the decrease in striatal TH^+ terminals after MPTP single dose, concluding that melatonin was able to prevent the damage caused by this drug in the striatal dopaminergic axons. In this way, Ortiz et al. [107] found apoptosis of the SNc dopaminergic neurons with an MPTP-unique dose; melatonin prevented cell death. Moreover, melatonin was able to avoid the reduction in striatal TH^+ immunoreactivity and the mitochondrial complex I alteration induced by 6-OHDA-lesion [108].

5. Conclusion

The results obtained in the present work provide evidence that melatonin pretreatment performs as a dopamine regulator protecting partially the striatal MSN dopaminergic denervation by preserving the dendritic spines and preventing the SNc TH^+ cell death, causing motor behavior recovery, as melatonin-pretreated mice displayed better motor performance and no parkinsonian symptoms, compared to Mn-exposed/no treatment mice.

It is likely that in the $MnCl_2/Mn(OAc)_3$ inhalation PD model, we are recreating an initial stage of the disease since the Mn-exposed mice lost ~70% of the dopaminergic cells, so we believe that it would be helpful to give melatonin to patients who start with the disease, in order to delay the symptoms and dopaminergic cell death and, above all, the start of L-DOPA treatment since it produces very disabling side effects for the patient.

Acknowledgements

This work was supported by COMECyT FICDTEM-2021-066 and PAPIIT-DGAPA IN216821 grants. We are very grateful to Veronica Rodriguez Mata for her excellent photographic and technical assistance.

Conflict of interest

Authors have declared that no competing interests exist.

Author details

Maria Rosa Avila-Costa[1*], Mariana Stephania Rodríguez-Alcántara[1], Ana Luisa Gutierréz-Valdez[1], José Luis Ordoñez-Librado[1], Vianey Rodríguez-Lara[2], Leonardo Reynoso-Erazo[3], Claudia Dorado-Martínez[1], Cesar Alfonso Garcia Caballero[1], Enrique Montiel-Flores[1], Javier Sanchez-Betancourt[1], Rocío Tron-Alvarez[3], Patricia Aley-Medina[1] and Jesús Espinosa-Villanueva[1]

1 Neuromorphology Lab, Facultad de Estudios Superiores Iztacala, UNAM, Tlalnepantla, Edo. Mex., Mexico

2 Department of Cell Biology, Faculty of Medicine, Nacional University of Mexico (UNAM), Mexico City, Mexico

3 Health Education Project, Facultad de Estudios Superiores Iztacala, UNAM, Tlalnepantla, Edo. Mex., Mexico

*Address all correspondence to: nigraizo@unam.mx; avila_costa@me.com

References

[1] Willis AW. Parkinson disease in the elderly adult. Missouri Medicine. 2013;**110**:406-410

[2] Schapira AH. Recent developments in biomarkers in Parkinson disease. Current Opinion in Neurology. 2013;**26**:395-400. DOI: 10.1097/WCO.0b013e3283633741

[3] Khandhar SM, Marks WJ. Epidemiology of Parkinson's disease. Disease-a-Month. 2007;**53**:200-205. DOI: 10.1016/j.disamonth.2007.02.001

[4] Alexander GE. Biology of Parkinson's disease: Pathogenesis and pathophysiology of a multisystem neurodegenerative disorder. Dialogues in Clinical Neuroscience. 2004;**6**:259-280. DOI: 10.31887/DCNS.2004.6.3/galexander

[5] Ross GW, Petrovitch H, Abbott RD, Nelson J, Markesbery W, Davis D, et al. Parkinsonian signs and substantia nigra neuron density in decendents elders without PD. Annals of Neurology. 2004;**56**:532-539. DOI: 10.1002/ana.20226

[6] Conway KA, Rochet JC, Bieganski RM, Lansbury PT. Kinetic stabilization of the alpha-synuclein protofibril by a dopamine-alpha-synuclein adduct. Science. 2001;**294**:1346-1349. DOI: 10.1126/science.1063522

[7] Büeler H. Impaired mitochondrial dynamics and function in the pathogenesis of Parkinson's disease. Experimental Neurology. 2009;**218**:235-246. DOI: 10.1016/j.expneurol.2009.03.006

[8] Barzilai A, Melamed E. Molecular mechanisms of selective dopaminergic neuronal death in Parkinson's disease. Trends in Molecular Medicine. 2003;**9**:126-132. DOI: 10.1016/s1471-4914(03)00020-0

[9] Toulouse A, Sullivan AM. Progress in Parkinson's disease-where do we stand? Progress in Neurobiology. 2008;**85**:376-392. DOI: 10.1016/j.pneurobio.2008.05.003

[10] Jankovic J. Parkinson's disease and movement disorders: Moving forward. Lancet Neurology. 2008;**7**:9-11. DOI: 10.1016/S1474-4422(07)70302-2

[11] Terzioglu M, Galter D. Parkinson's disease: Genetic versus toxin-induced rodent models. The FEBS Journal. 2008;**275**:1384-1391. DOI: 10.1111/j.1742-4658.2008.06302.x

[12] Hernandez DG, Reed X, Singleton AB. Genetics in Parkinson disease: Mendelian versus non-Mendelian inheritance. Journal of Neurochemistry. 2016;**139**(Suppl 1):59-74. DOI: 10.1111/jnc.13593

[13] Betarbet R, Sherer TB, Greenamyre JT. Animal models of Parkinson's disease. BioEssays. 2002;**24**:308-318. DOI: 10.1002/bies.10067

[14] Greenamyre JT, Betarbet R, Sherer TB. The rotenone model of Parkinson's disease: Genes, environment and mitochondria. Parkinsonism & Related Disorders. 2003;**9**(Suppl 2):S59-S64. DOI: 10.1016/s1353-8020(03)00023-3

[15] Kalia LV, Lang AE. Parkinson's disease. Lancet. 2015;**386**:896-912. DOI: 10.1016/S0140-6736(14)61393-3

[16] Ferreira M, Massano J. An updated review of Parkinson's disease genetics and clinicopathological correlations.

Acta Neurologica Scandinavica. 2017;**135**: 273-284. DOI: 10.1111/ane.12616

[17] Polymeropoulos MH, Lavedan C, Leroy E, Ide SE, Dehejia A, Dutra A, et al. Mutation in the alpha-synuclein gene identified in families with Parkinson's disease. Science. 1997;**276**:2045-2047. DOI: 10.1126/science.276.5321.2045

[18] Fahn S, Cohen G. The oxidant stress hypothesis in Parkinson's disease: Evidence supporting it. Annals of Neurology. 1992;**32**:804-812. DOI: 10.1002/ana.410320616

[19] Jenner P, Olanow CW. Oxidative stress and the pathogenesis of Parkinson's disease. Neurology. 1996;**47**:161-170. DOI: 10.1212/wnl.47.6_suppl_3.161s

[20] Taylor JM, Main BS, Crack PJ. Neuroinflammation and oxidative stress: Co-conspirators in the pathology of Parkinson's disease. Neurochemistry International. 2013;**62**:803-819. DOI: 10.1016/j.neuint.2012.12.016

[21] Trushina E, McMurray CT. Oxidative stress and mitochondrial dysfunction in neurodegenerative diseases. Neuroscience. 2007;**145**:1233-1248. DOI: 10.1016/j.neuroscience.2006.10.056

[22] Ebadi M, Srinivasan SK, Baxi MD. Oxidative stress and antioxidant therapy in Parkinson's disease. Progress in Neurobiology. 1996;**48**:1-19. DOI: 10.1016/0301-0082(95)00029-1

[23] Ebadi M, Govitrapong P, Sharma S, Muralikrishnan D, Shavali S, Pellett L, et al. Ubiquinone (coenzyme q10) and mitochondria in oxidative stress of Parkinson's disease. Biological Signals and Receptors. 2001;**10**:224-253. DOI: 10.1159/000046889

[24] Bove J, Prou D, Perier C, Przedborski S. Toxin-induced models of Parkinson's disease. NeuroRx. 2005;**2**:484-494. DOI: 10.1602/neurorx.2.3.484

[25] Schober A. Classic toxin-induced animal models of Parkinson's disease: 6-OHDA and MPTP. Cell and Tissue Research. 2004;**318**:215-224. DOI: 10.1007/s00441-004-0938-y

[26] Ordoñez-Librado JL, Anaya-Martínez V, Gutierrez-Valdez AL, Colín-Barenque L, Montiel-Flores E, Avila-Costa MR. Manganese inhalation as a Parkinson disease model. Parkinson's Disease. 2010;**2011**:612989. DOI: 10.4061/2011/612989

[27] Ordoñez-Librado JL, Gutierrez-Valdez AL, Colín-Barenque L, Anaya-Martínez V, Díaz-Bech P, Avila-Costa MR. Inhalation of divalent and trivalent manganese mixture induces a Parkinson's disease model: Immunocytochemical and behavioral evidences. Neuroscience. 2008;**155**:7-16. DOI: 10.1016/j.neuroscience.2008.05.012

[28] Sánchez-Betancourt J, Anaya-Martínez V, Gutiérrez-Valdez AL, Ordóñez-Librado JL, Montiel-Flores E, Espinosa-Villanueva J, et al. Manganese mixture inhalation is a reliable Parkinson disease model in rats. Neurotoxicology. 2012;**33**:1346-1355. DOI: 10.1016/j.neuro.2012.08.012

[29] Ordoñez-Librado JL, Anaya-Martinez V, Gutierrez-Valdez AL, Montiel-Flores E, Corona DR, Martinez-Fong D, et al. L-DOPA treatment reverses the motor alterations induced by manganese exposure as a Parkinson disease experimental model. Neuroscience Letters. 2010;**471**:79-82. DOI: 10.1016/j.neulet.2010.01.015

[30] Rascol O, Brooks DJ, Korczyn AD, PPd D, Clarke CE, Lang AE. A five-year study of the incidence of dyskinesia in

patients with early Parkinson's disease who were treated with ropinirole or levodopa. New England Journal of Medicine. 2000;**342**:1484-1491. DOI: 10.1056/NEJM200005183422004

[31] Lang AE, Lozano AM. Parkinson's disease. First of two parts. New England Journal of Medicine. 1998;**339**:1044-1053. DOI: 10.1056/NEJM199810083391506

[32] Lang AE, Lozano AM. Parkinson's disease. Second of two parts. New England Journal of Medicine. 1998;**339**:1130-1143. DOI: 10.1056/NEJM199810153391607

[33] Rascol O, Payoux P, Ory F, Ferreira JJ, Brefel-Courbon C, Montastruc JL. Limitations of current Parkinson's disease therapy. Annals of Neurology. 2003;**53**(Suppl 3):S3-S12; discussion S-5. DOI: 10.1002/ana.10513

[34] Beck KD, Valverde J, Alexi T, Poulsen K, Moffat B, Vandlen RA, et al. Mesencephalic dopaminergic neurons protected by GDNF from axotomy-induced degeneration in the adult brain. Nature. 1995;**373**:339-341. DOI: 10.1038/373339a0

[35] Tassigny XA, Pascual A, López-Barneo J. GDNF-based therapies, GDNF-producing interneurons, and trophic support of the dopaminergic nigrostriatal pathway. Implications for Parkinson's disease. Frontiers in Neuroanatomy. 2015;**9**:10. DOI: 10.3389/fnana.2015.00010

[36] van Hilten JJ, Ramaker C, Van de Beek WJ, Finken MJ. Bromocriptine for levodopa-induced motor complications in Parkinson's disease. Cochrane Database of Systematic Reviews. 2000;**2**:CD001203. DOI: 10.1002/14651858.CD001203

[37] Ramaker C, van de Beek WJ, Finken MJ, van Hilten BJ. The efficacy and safety of adjunct bromocriptine therapy for levodopa-induced motor complications: A systematic review. Movement Disorders. 2000;**15**: 56-64. DOI: 10.1002/1531-8257(200001)15:1<56::aid-mds1010>3.0.co;2-2

[38] Avila-Costa MR, Colin-Barenque L, Montiel-Flores E, Aley-Medina P, Valdez AL, Librado JL, et al. Bromocriptine treatment in a murine Parkinson's model: Ultrastructural evaluation after dopaminergic deafferentation. The International Journal of Neuroscience. 2005;**115**:851-859. DOI: 10.1080/00207450590897059

[39] Boyd A. Bromocriptine and psychosis: A literature review. The Psychiatric Quarterly. 1995;**66**:87-95. DOI: 10.1007/BF02238717

[40] Radad K, Gille G, Rausch WD. Short review on dopamine agonists: Insight into clinical and research studies relevant to Parkinson's disease. Pharmacological Reports. 2005;**57**:701-712

[41] Chen JJ, Obering C. A review of intermittent subcutaneous apomorphine injections for the rescue management of motor fluctuations associated with advanced Parkinson's disease. Clinical Therapeutics. 2005;**27**:1710-1724. DOI: 10.1016/j.clinthera.2005.11.016

[42] Piercey MF. Pharmacology of pramipexole, a dopamine D3-preferring agonist useful in treating Parkinson's disease. Clinical Neuropharmacology. 1998;**21**:141-151

[43] Linazasoro G, Spanish Dopamine Agonists Study G. Conversion from dopamine agonists to pramipexole. An open-label trial in 227 patients with advanced Parkinson's disease. Journal of Neurology. 2004;**251**:335-339. DOI: 10.1007/s00415-004-0328-0

[44] Brusa L, Bassi A, Stefani A, Pierantozzi M, Peppe A, Caramia MD, et al. Pramipexole in comparison to l-dopa: A neuropsychological study. Journal of Neural Transmission (Vienna). 2003;**110**:373-380. DOI: 10.1007/s00702-002-0811-7

[45] Lipski J, Nistico R, Berretta N, Guatteo E, Bernardi G, Mercuri NB. L-DOPA: A scapegoat for accelerated neurodegeneration in Parkinson's disease? Progress in Neurobiology. 2011;**94**:389-407. DOI: 10.1016/j.pneurobio.2011.06.005

[46] Mercuri NB, Bernardi G. The 'magic' of L-dopa: Why is it the gold standard Parkinson's disease therapy? Trends in Pharmacological Sciences. 2005;**26**:341-344. DOI: 10.1016/j.tips.2005.05.002

[47] Picconi B, Paille V, Ghiglieri V, Bagetta V, Barone I, Lindgren HS, et al. L-DOPA dosage is critically involved in dyskinesia via loss of synaptic depotentiation. Neurobiology of Disease. 2008;**29**:327-335. DOI: 10.1016/j.nbd.2007.10.001

[48] Calabresi P, Filippo MD, Ghiglieri V, Tambasco N, Picconi B. Levodopa-induced dyskinesias in patients with Parkinson's disease: Filling the bench-to-bedside gap. Lancet Neurology. 2010;**9**:1106-1117. DOI: 10.1016/S1474-4422(10)70218-0

[49] Whetten-Goldstein K, Sloan F, Kulas E, Cutson T, Schenkman M. The burden of Parkinson's disease on society, family, and the individual. Journal of the American Geriatrics Society. 1997;**45**:844-849. DOI: 10.1111/j.1532-5415.1997.tb01512.x

[50] Rao G, Xia E, Richardson A. Effect of age on the expression of antioxidant enzymes in male Fischer F344 rats. Mechanisms of Ageing and Development. 1990;**53**:49-60. DOI: 10.1016/0047-6374(90)90033-c

[51] Sen CK, Khanna S, Roy S. Tocotrienol: The natural vitamin E to defend the nervous system? Annals of the New York Academy of Sciences. 2004;**1031**:127-142. DOI: 10.1196/annals.1331.013

[52] Singh S, Ahmed R, Sagar RK, Krishana B. Neuroprotection of the nigrostriatal dopaminergic neurons by melatonin in hemiparkinsonium rat. The Indian Journal of Medical Research. 2006;**124**:419-426

[53] Ali SF, Imam SZ, Itzhak Y. Role of peroxynitrite in methamphetamine-induced dopaminergic neurodegeneration and neuroprotection by antioxidants and selective NOS inhibitors. Annals of the New York Academy of Sciences. 2005;**1053**:97-98. DOI: 10.1196/annals.1344.053

[54] Bonnefont-Rousselot D, Collin F. Melatonin: Action as antioxidant and potential applications in human disease and aging. Toxicology. 2010;**278**:55-67. DOI: 10.1016/j.tox.2010.04.008

[55] Gutiérrez-Valdez AL, Anaya-Martínez V, Ordóñez-Librado JL, García-Ruiz R, Torres-Esquivel C, Moreno-Rivera M, et al. Effect of chronic L-Dopa or melatonin treatments after dopamine deafferentation in rats: Dyskinesia, motor performance, and cytological analysis. ISRN Neurology. 2012;**2012**:1-16. DOI: 10.5402/2012/360379

[56] Hardeland R, Cardinali DP, Srinivasan V, Spence DW, Brown GM, Pandi-Perumal SR. Melatonin—A pleiotropic, orchestrating regulator molecule. Progress in Neurobiology. 2011;**93**:350-384. DOI: 10.1016/j.pneurobio.2010.12.004

[57] Hardeland R, Pandi-Perumal SR, Cardinali DP. Melatonin. The International Journal of Biochemistry & Cell Biology. 2006;**38**(3):313-316. DOI: 10.1016/j.biocel.2005.08.020

[58] Tan DX, Manchester LC, Hardeland R, Lopez-Burillo S, Mayo JC, Sainz RM, et al. Melatonin: A hormone, a tissue factor, an autocoid, a paracoid, and an antioxidant vitamin. Journal of Pineal Research. 2003;**34**:75-78. DOI: 10.1034/j.1600-079x.2003.02111.x

[59] Hardeland R, Pandi-Perumal SR. Melatonin, a potent agent in antioxidative defense: Actions as a natural food constituent, gastrointestinal factor, drug and prodrug. Nutrition and Metabolism. 2005;**2**:22. DOI: 10.1186/1743-7075-2-22

[60] Pinol-Ripoll G, Fuentes-Broto L, Millan-Plano S, Reyes-Gonzales M, Mauri JA, Martinez-Ballarin E, et al. Protective effect of melatonin and pinoline on nitric oxide-induced lipid and protein peroxidation in rat brain homogenates. Neuroscience Letters. 2006;**405**:89-93. DOI: 10.1016/j.neulet.2006.06.031

[61] Kundurovic Z, Sofic E. The effects of exogenous Melatonin on the morphology of thyrocytes in pinealectomized and irradiated rats. Journal of Neural Transmission. 2006;**113**:49-58. DOI: 10.1007/s00702-005-0396-z

[62] Dubocovich ML, Delagrange P, Krause DN, Sugden D, Cardinali DP, Olcese J. International Union of Basic and Clinical Pharmacology. LXXV. Nomenclature, classification, and pharmacology of G protein-coupled melatonin receptors. Pharmacological Reviews. 2010;**62**:343-380. DOI: 10.1124/pr.110.002832

[63] Srinivasan V, Pandi-Perumal SR, Cardinali DP, Poeggeler B, Hardeland R. Melatonin in Alzheimer's disease and other neurodegenerative disorders. Behavioral and brain functions. Behavioral and Brain Functions. 2006;**2**:15. DOI: 10.1186/1744-9081-2-15

[64] Feeney Dennis M, Gonzalez A, Law WA. Amphetamine, haloperidol, and experience interact to affect rate of recovery after motor cortex injury. Science. 1982;**217**:855-857. DOI: 10.1126/science.7100929

[65] Farr TD, Whishaw IQ. Quantitative and qualitative impairments in skilled reaching in the mouse (*Mus musculus*) after a focal motor cortex stroke. Stroke. 2002;**33**:1869-1875. DOI: 10.1161/01.str.0000020714.48349.4e

[66] Avila-Costa MR, Montiel Flores E, Colin-Barenque L, Ordoñez JL, Gutiérrez AL, Niño-Cabrera HG, et al. Nigrostriatal modifications after vanadium inhalation: An immunocytochemical and cytological approach. Neurochemical Research. 2004;**29**:1365-1369. DOI: 10.1023/b:nere.0000026398.86113.7d

[67] Valverde F. The golgi method. A tool for comparative structural analyses. In: WJH N, SOE E, editors. Contemporary Research Methods in Neuroanatomy. Berlin, Heidelberg: Springer Berlin Heidelberg; 1970. pp. 12-31. DOI: 10.1007/978-3-642-85986-1_2

[68] Lloyd KG, Davidson L, Hornykiewicz O. The neurochemistry of Parkinson's disease: Effect of L-dopa therapy. The Journal of Pharmacology and Experimental Therapeutics. 1975;**195**:453-464

[69] Alexander GE, Crutcher MD, DeLong MR. Basal ganglia-thalamocortical circuits: Parallel substrates for motor, oculomotor, "prefrontal" and

"limbic" functions. Progress in Brain Research. 1990;**85**:119-146

[70] Elble RJ, Cousins R, Leffler K, Hughes L. Gait initiation by patients with lower-half parkinsonism. Brain. 1996;**119**:1705-1716. DOI: 10.1093/brain/119.5.1705

[71] Morris ME, Iansek R, Matyas TA, Summers JJ. The pathogenesis of gait hypokinesia in Parkinson's disease. Brain. 1994;**117**:1169-1181. DOI: 10.1093/brain/117.5.1169

[72] Morris M, Iansek R, Matyas T, Summers J. Abnormalities in the stride length-cadence relation in parkinsonian gait. Movement Disorders. 1998;**13**:61-69. DOI: 10.1002/mds.870130115

[73] Blin O, Ferrandez AM, Serratrice G. Quantitative analysis of gait in Parkinson patients: Increased variability of stride length. Journal of the Neurological Sciences. 1990;**98**:91-97. DOI: 10.1016/0022-510x(90)90184-o

[74] Fernagut PO, Diguet E, Labattu B, Tison F. A simple method to measure stride length as an index of nigrostriatal dysfunction in mice. Journal of Neuroscience Methods. 2002;**113**:123-130. DOI: 10.1016/s0165-0270(01)00485-x

[75] Tan D-x, Manchester LC, Reiter RJ, Qi W, Hanes MA, Farley NJ. High physiological levels of melatonin in the bile of mammals. Life Sciences. 1999;**65**:2523-2529. DOI: 10.1016/s0024-3205(99)00519-6

[76] Reiter RJ, Tan D-x, Terron MP, Flores LJ, Czarnocki Z. Melatonin and its metabolites: New findings regarding their production and their radical scavenging actions. Acta Biochimica Polonica. 2007;**54**:1-9

[77] Whishaw IQ, Pellis SM, Gorny BP, Pellis VC. The impairments in reaching and the movements of compensation in rats with motor cortex lesions: An endpoint, videorecording, and movement notation analysis. Behavioural Brain Research. 1991;**42**:77-91. DOI: 10.1016/s0166-4328(05)80042-7

[78] Whishaw IQ, Suchowersky O, Davis L, Sarna J, Metz GA, Pellis SM. Impairment of pronation, supination, and body coordination in reach-to-grasp tasks in human Parkinson's disease (PD) reveals homology to deficits in animal models. Behavioural Brain Research. 2002;**133**:165-176. DOI: 10.1016/s0166-4328(01)00479-x

[79] Castiello U, Bennett K, Bonfiglioli C, Lim S, Peppard FR. The reach-to-grasp movement in Parkinson's disease: Response to a simultaneous perturbation of object position and object size. Experimental Brain Research. 1999;**125**(4):453-462

[80] Anaya-Martínez V, Gutiérrez-Valdez AL, Ordóñez-Librado JL, Sanchez-Betancourt J, Montiel-Flores E, Reynoso-Erazo L, et al. L-DOPA/melatonin combination as an alternative Parkinson disease treatment. Current Trends in Neurology. 2015;**8**:87-104. ISSN: 0972-8252

[81] Cordova FM, Aguiar AS, Peres TV, Lopes MW, Gonçalves FM, Pedro DZ, et al. Manganese-exposed developing rats display motor deficits and striatal oxidative stress that are reversed by Trolox. Archives of Toxicology. 2013;**87**:1231-1244. DOI: 10.1007/s00204-013-1017-5

[82] Fernsebner K, Zorn J, Kanawati B, Walker A, Michalke B. Manganese leads to an increase in markers of oxidative stress as well as to a shift in the ratio of

Fe(ii)/(iii) in rat brain tissue. Metallomics. 2014;**6**:921-931. DOI: 10.1039/c4mt00022f

[83] Erikson KM, Dobson AW, Dorman DC, Aschner M. Manganese exposure and induced oxidative stress in the rat brain. Science of the Total Environment. 2004;**334-335**:409-416. DOI: 10.1016/j.scitotenv.2004.04.044

[84] Deng Y, Jiao C, Mi C, Xu B, Li Y, Wang F, et al. Melatonin inhibits manganese-induced motor dysfunction and neuronal loss in mice: Involvement of oxidative stress and dopaminergic neurodegeneration. Molecular Neurobiology. 2014;**51**:68-88. DOI: 10.1007/s12035-014-8789-3

[85] Tomás-Zapico C, Coto-Montes A. A proposed mechanism to explain the stimulatory effect of melatonin on antioxidative enzymes. Journal of Pineal Research. 2005;**39**(2):99-104

[86] Avila-Costa M, Gutierrez-Valdez A, Ordonez-Librado J, Martinez V, Colin-Barenque L, Espinosa-Villanueva J, et al. Time course changes of the striatum neuropil after unilateral dopamine depletion and the usefulness of the contralateral striatum as a control structure. Neurological Research. 2008;**30**:1068-1074. DOI: 10.1179/174313208X346116

[87] Villalba RM, Lee H, Smith Y. Dopaminergic denervation and spine loss in the striatum of MPTP-treated monkeys. Experimental Neurology. 2009;**215**:220-227. DOI: 10.1016/j.expneurol.2008.09.025

[88] Zaja-Milatovic S, Milatovic D, Schantz AM, Zhang J, Montine KS, Samii A, et al. Dendritic degeneration in neostriatal medium spiny neurons in Parkinson disease. Neurology. 2005;**64**:545-547. DOI: 10.1212/01.WNL.0000150591.33787.A4

[89] Archibald FS, Tyree C. Manganese poisoning and the attack of trivalent manganese upon catecholamines. Archives of Biochemistry and Biophysics. 1987;**256**:638-650. DOI: 10.1016/0003-9861(87)90621-7

[90] Ingham CAHS, Taggart P, Arbuthnott GW. Plasticity of synapses in the rat neostriatum after unilateral lesion of the nigrostriatal dopaminergic pathway. The Journal of Neuroscience. 1998;**15**:4732-4743. DOI: 10.1523/JNEUROSCI.18-12-04732.1998

[91] Cavazos JE, Golarai G, Sutula TP. Mossy fiber synaptic reorganization induced by kindling: Time course of development, progression, and permanence. The Journal of Neuroscience. 1991;**11**:2795-2803. DOI: 10.1523/JNEUROSCI.11-09-02795.1991

[92] Day M, Wang Z, Ding J, An X, Ingham CA, Shering AF, et al. Selective elimination of glutamatergic synapses on striatopallidal neurons in Parkinson disease models. Nature Neuroscience. 2006;**9**:251-259. DOI: 10.1038/nn1632

[93] Gerfen CR. Indirect-pathway neurons lose their spines in Parkinson disease. Nature Neuroscience. 2006;**9**:157-158. DOI: 10.1038/nn0206-157

[94] Küçükkaya B, Haklar G, Yalçin AS. NMDA excitotoxicity and free radical generation in rat brain homogenates: Application of a chemiluminescence assay. Neurochemical Research. 1996;**21**:1535-1538. DOI: 10.1007/BF02533102

[95] Reiter RJ, Tan DX, Osuna C, Gitto E. Actions of melatonin in the reduction of oxidative stress. A review. Journal of Biomedical Science. 2000;**7**:444-458. DOI: 10.1007/BF02253360

[96] Smith Y, Raju D, Nanda B, Pare JF, Galvan A, Wichmann T. The thalamostriatal

systems: Anatomical and functional organization in normal and parkinsonian states. Brain Research Bulletin. 2009;**78**:60-68. DOI: 10.1016/j.brainresbull.2008.08.015

[97] Damier P, Hirsch EC, Agid Y, Graybiel AM. The substantia nigra of the human brain. I. Nigrosomes and the nigral matrix, a compartmental organization based on calbindin D(28K) immunohistochemistry. Brain. 1999;**122**:1421-1436. DOI: 10.1093/brain/122.8.1421

[98] Allbutt HN, Henderson JM. Use of the narrow beam test in the rat, 6-hydroxydopamine model of Parkinson's disease. Journal of Neuroscience Methods. 2007;**159**:195-202. DOI: 10.1016/j.jneumeth.2006.07.006

[99] Dowd E, Dunnett SB. Comparison of 6-hydroxydopamine-induced medial forebrain bundle and nigrostriatal terminal lesions in a lateralised nose-poking task in rats. Behavioural Brain Research. 2005;**159**:153-161. DOI: 10.1016/j.bbr.2004.10.010

[100] Erikson KM, John CE, Jones SR, Aschner M. Manganese accumulation in striatum of mice exposed to toxic doses is dependent upon a functional dopamine transporter. Environmental Toxicology and Pharmacology. 2005;**20**:390-394. DOI: 10.1016/j.etap.2005.03.009

[101] Calne DB, Chu NS, Huang CC, Lu CS, Olanow W. Manganism and idiopathic parkinsonism: Similarities and differences. Neurology. 1994;**44**:1583-1586. DOI: 10.1212/wnl.44.9.1583

[102] Zhang S, Fu J, Zhou Z. In vitro effect of manganese chloride exposure on reactive oxygen species generation and respiratory chain complexes activities of mitochondria isolated from rat brain. Toxicology In Vitro. 2004;**18**:71-77. DOI: 10.1016/j.tiv.2003.09.002

[103] Leon J, Acuna-Castroviejo D, Escames G, Tan DX, Reiter RJ. Melatonin mitigates mitochondrial malfunction. Journal of Pineal Research. 2005;**38**:1-9. DOI: 10.1111/j.1600-079X.2004.00181.x

[104] Morcillo P, Cordero H, Ijomone OM, Ayodele A, Bornhorst J, Gunther L, et al. Defective mitochondrial dynamics underlie manganese-induced neurotoxicity. Molecular Neurobiology. 2021;**58**:3270-3289. DOI: 10.1007/s12035-021-02341-w

[105] Antolin I, Mayo JC, Sainz RM, del Brio ML, Herrera F, Martin V, et al. Protective effect of melatonin in a chronic experimental model of Parkinson's disease. Brain Research. 2002;**943**:163-173. DOI: 10.1016/s0006-8993(02)02551-9

[106] Acuña-Castroviejo D, Coto-Montes A, Gaia Monti M, Ortiz GG, Reiter RJ. Melatonin is protective against MPTP-induced striatal and hippocampal lesions. Life Sciences. 1997;**60**:PL23-PL29. DOI: 10.1016/s0024-3205(96)00606-6

[107] Ortiz GG, Crespo-López ME, Morán-Moguel C, García JJ, Reiter RJ, Acuña-Castroviejo D. Protective role of melatonin against MPTP-induced mouse brain cell DNA fragmentation and apoptosis in vivo. Neuro Endocrinology Letters. 2001;**22**:101-108

[108] Dabbeni-Sala F, Di Santo S, Franceschini D, Skaper SD, Giusti P. Melatonin protects against 6-OHDA-induced neurotoxicity in rats: A role for mitochondrial complex I activity. The FASEB Journal. 2001;**15**:164-170. DOI: 10.1096/fj.00-0129com

Section 5

Melatonin as a Feed Additive

Chapter 7

Use of Melatonin as a Feed Additive

Oğuzhan Kahraman, Zekeriya Safa İnanç, Huzur Derya Arık and Mustafa Selçuk Alataş

Abstract

Melatonin is a molecule that plays an active role in reducing many stress factors in plants and has important functions in the growth, development and reproduction of plants. It has many physiological functions that directly affect feed consumption, feed efficiency, energy metabolism and immune system in animal organisms. In addition, its anti-inflammatory, antioxidant, anticancer and antiapoptotic effects are also known. While melatonin has an antioxidative effect at low doses, it can exert a prooxidant effect at high doses. It has been suggested that when melatonin is used as a silage additive, it increases the total acid content of the silage and significantly improves the silage fermentation quality by lowering the pH level and butyric acid. Although it has positive effects on mammary gland involution and general health in ruminants, its effects on yield parameters have not been proven. Broilers and layers are expected high productivity and performance, in this regard, they are faced with stress factors such as intensive feeding and housing conditions. Considering its positive effects on stress factors, health and productivity, melatonin is a promising feed additive. Effects of melatonin additive or supplements on animal productivity and health should be revealed in further studies.

Keywords: additive, melatonin, poultry, ruminant

1. Introduction

Melatonin is recognized as an active oxygen scavenger, which can inhibit peroxidation, effectively scavenge reactive oxygen radicals, delay the wilting of plants, and alleviate salt, drought, heavy metal, cold, pathogens and other adversities [1]. Melatonin, a derivative of tryptophan, has a low molecular weight and an indole ring structure and is an evolutionarily conserved pleiotropic molecule ubiquitous in living organisms. Melatonin is a molecule that plays an active role in reducing many stress factors in plants and has important functions in the growth, development and reproduction of plants [2]. It is accepted that melatonin can regulate vegetative growth and flowering processes such as rooting, photosynthetic yield and biomass yield, and plays a potential regulator role in the formation and maturation of fruits and seeds [3].

Melatonin is a substance secreted by the pineal gland in the darkness and can regulate biological rhythms in many physiological systems in animals, including the behavioral, cardiovascular, reproductive, immune, excretory, thermoregulatory and neuroendocrine systems [4]. Melatonin has many physiological functions that directly affects feed consumption, feed efficiency, energy metabolism and immune system in animals. Studies on the effects of melatonin on animals have shown different results [5, 6]. In a study on the use of melatonin as a silage additive, Li et al. stated that it significantly improved the quality of the silage by increased volatile fatty acid levels and decreased pH. In addition to these positive effects, melatonin had curative effects on silage fermentation by increasing microbial diversity [1].

The use of melatonin as an additive is not common. Because, melatonin has not been studied sufficiently in animals as a feed additive and its effects have not been adequately explained. In this chapter, the effects of melatonin as a feed additive especially in ruminants, broiler and layer chickens on production, yield and animal health were reviewed in order to popularize the use of melatonin as an additive and supplement. Also, the effects and functions of melatonin on plants were tried to be explained.

2. Synthesis and functional properties of melatonin in animals

Melatonin was isolated from the pituitary gland in 1958. A lot of research has been conducted about the effects and usage areas of melatonin. It was discovered as a skin lightening molecule that acts on frog and fish melanocytes, and found to be an important hormone rhythmically secreted by the brain's pineal gland [7, 8]. The relationship between the pineal gland and light has caused it to be called the third eye. Melatonin can be synthesized in almost every living creatures, including many vertebrates and invertebrates, bacteria, protozoa, plants and fungi. Melatonin has immunostimulatory and cytoprotective agent functions that regulate the sleep-wake cycle. Also, it activates T and B lymphocytes, monocytes and stimulates the reproduction of thymocyte cells and the release of cytokines. In addition to these, its anti-inflammatory, antioxidant, anticancer and antiapoptotic effects are also known [9].

Apart from the pineal gland, melatonin is also secreted from the ovary, lens of the eye, bone marrow cells, gall bladder and gastrointestinal tract. However, the level of circulating melatonin reflects the production of melatonin in the pineal gland. While there is no difference in terms of human and animal health in matters such as the mode of action, release and chemical structure of melatonin, its usage areas vary. The antioxidant properties of melatonin and its effect on sleep disorders are at the forefront on humans. But, it has also been reported to have protective effects in neuronal degeneration and neuroprotective properties in oxidative stress-induced neuronal apoptosis [10, 11].

Light exposure level is the most effective factor that determines the rate of melatonin secretion. In general, light decreases melatonin production, while darkness increases it. The starting material of melatonin synthesis is tryptophan, an indole amino acid taken from plasma [12]. Tryptophan is hydroxylated to 5-hydroxytryptophan in pinealocytes by the enzyme tryptophanhydroxylase. 5-hydroxytryptophan is decarboxylated to 5-hydroxytryptamine (seratonin) by aromatic-L-amino acid decarboxylase. Seratonin is converted to N-acetylseratonin by N-acetyltransferase (NAT) enzyme, and this is converted to melatonin (N-acetyl-5-methoxytryptamine) by the effect of hydroxyindole-o-methyl transferase (HOMT). It has been determined that NAT and HOMT activities, which enable the conversion of serotonin to melatonin, are higher at night. It has been demonstrated by immunohistochemical methods that the enzymes required for melatonin synthesis are also present in the suprachiasmatic nucleus, retina and small intestine, apart from pinealocytes [13, 14].

After melatonin is synthesized in the pineal gland, it quickly passes into the capillaries without being stored in the organism. Due to its high lipophilic effect, it can be distributed to many biological tissues and fluids in the organism. Approximately 70% of plasma is transported bound to albumin. While melatonin can be metabolized in the kidney, this process generally takes place in the liver. Melatonin is converted to 6-hydroxymelatonin in the liver; this, in turn, binds to sulfate and glucuronic acid through the kidneys and is excreted in the urine [15].

Morphological, biochemical and molecular studies in both animals and humans in recent years have shown that oxidative stress plays a primary role in the development of degenerative changes in cells and tissues in our body. The highest degree of oxidative damage usually occurs in organs such as the brain, heart, and skeletal muscle. Melatonin inhibits free radicals from their pyrrole rings and interacts with them, reducing their activity. It also shows its effect by inducing the production of antioxidants. Melatonin has the ability to scavenge all free radicals formed in the cell. Thus, an increase is observed in the expression of genes encoding antioxidants, while genes that cause an increase in free radicals are suppressed metabolites such as melatonin also have very protective effects against oxidative stress. Lipid peroxidation, which occurs as a result of oxidative damage and accumulation of free radicals in cells, causes deterioration in cell membranes. As a result of damage, signal transmission and activation of signal pathways in cells are affected and various metabolic functions become ineffective. Melatonin prevents this lipid peroxidation and minimizes cell damage. Melatonin also neutralizes radicals caused by nitrogen and prevents nitric oxide formed [16].

3. Effects of melatonin in plants

Under extreme stress conditions, the natural defense mechanisms of plants do not provide adequate protection; In this case, exogenous biostimulants can be used to improve plant stress tolerance [17]. Recent studies have indicated that plant growth regulators manage stress mechanisms. Among these regulators, melatonin (N-acetyl-5-methoxytryptamine) is a functional natural antioxidant widely used among plants [18]. While melatonin plays an important role in plant growth and development, it promotes root and hypocotyl growth and increases the biomass of plants with its auxin-like functions [19]. Studies on the functions of melatonin in plants have revealed that melatonin plays a very important role in plant growth and development under abiotic stress conditions. Melatonin is known to increase plant tolerance under salinity stress, improve photosynthesis capacity to maintain plant ionic balance ($Na+/K+$ ratio), protect chlorophyll and carotenoids, and reduce photorespiration [1]. The transcriptome analysis results showed that melatonin particularly affected the pathways of plant hormone signal transduction and biosynthesis of secondary metabolites.

Melatonin is a powerful antioxidant and has the ability to purify reactive oxygen species, reactive nitrogen species and various chemical pollutants. It has been suggested that melatonin detoxifies the oxidative stress caused by excess cadmium in tomatoes by stimulating antioxidant enzymatic activity [20]. In another study, it was reported that antioxidants suppress H_2O_2 production, reduce malondialdehyde and regulate various physiological processes. In addition, exogenous application of melatonin improves the chlorophyll content and photosynthesis capacity of various plant species under salt stress by decreasing the production of reactive oxygen species and increasing the soluble protein content [21].

4. Use of melatonin as silage and feed additive in ruminants

Fresh roughage is fermented to preserve its nutrient content for a long time by ensiling. The purpose of silage additives is to control the fermentation products by ensuring domination of lactic acid bacteria during fermentation and to preserve the nutrients in the feed as much as possible. In recent years, the popularity of silage additives has increased and has found a wide range of uses. Many additives have been studied for many years to support the fermentation process. Additives improve feed consumption, feed efficiency and performance in animals with their positive effects on silage quality together with an efficient ensiling [22]. Many silage additives are produced biotechnologically. Among them, bacterial inoculants and enzymes are used to provide fast and effective silage fermentation. The purpose of using melatonin as an additive is to control silage fermentation, form the desired end products and obtain appropriate quality silage. Melatonin has antioxidant and bacteriostasis properties as a natural preservative. With these properties, it can be considered as a silage additive. There is no literature on the use of melatonin as an additive in corn or mazie silages used in dairy cattle feeding. However, *Stylosanthes guianensis* (stylo), one of the hot season legume forage plants, was ensiled with the addition of melatonin at different rates (5, 10, 20 mg/kg), and the rate of 5 mg/kg increased the lactic acid and total acid level, decreasing the pH value and butyric acid content. It was revealed that the silage fermentation quality was significantly improved. With its antioxidation effect, it inhibited unwanted bacteria and managed to protect the silage [23]. Melatonin is a promising silage additive as it improves the silage properties of one of the legume feeds, which is difficult to ensilage due to its high buffer capacity and low sugar content. It affected the silage microbiota and metabolism of the stylo plant [23]. There is insufficient literature on its use as a silage additive in various plants. The effects of melatonin on the quality of silage feeds, which are most commonly used in ruminant feeding, should be investigated by comparing them with other additives.

Cessation of milking initiates the dry period in dairy cattle, but milk production continues and begins to accumulate in the mammary. With accumulation, milk leaks may occur. In this case, the mammary becomes open to infection. Cows are at high risk of developing intramammary infections due to udder enlargement and altered immune functions during the transition period. When the mammary gland is completely involved, it becomes more resistant to infections. Therefore, it is beneficial to suppress milk yield and accelerate the involution process before the dry period [24]. The melatonin hormone is physiologically secreted at nights in cows. It has been determined that there is a higher rate of melatonin in milk in the morning. While prolonged exposure to sunlight is beneficial for lactating animals, it should be the opposite for animals in dry period. Exposure to sunlight for a short time or administration of melatonin during late lactation may accelerate mammary gland involution by reducing milk yield before the dry period. Several studies have found that the addition of melatonin to feed reduces blood prolactin levels. For example, the addition of melatonin at a dose of 4 mg/kg BW decreased the prolactin level in prepubertal heifers [25]. It has been reported that prolactin level decreased with the addition of melatonin to the rations of cows in the late lactation period for 8 weeks. However, melatonin mixed into the ration did not affect milk yield [26]. It has been reported that the application of melatonin in the form of implants without mixing with the feed did not affect the milk yield of the cows in the postpartum period [27].

The effect of melatonin feeding on prolactin hormone in prepartum heifers and cows was not as effective as "short day photoperiod" (SDPP, 16 s dark-8 s light) application [24]. The positive effects of melatonin supplementation in prepartum period on milk production in postpartum period are not certain. This may also be related to short trial duration or insufficient number of cows. Lacasse et al. applied "long day photoperiod" (LDPP, 16 s light-8 s dark) to cows starting 8 weeks before calving and added 25 mg melatonin to feed. It was stated that the milk yield of the cows treated with SDPP in the early lactation period was higher than those treated with LDPP + melatonin [28]. This situation can be explained by the source of the melatonin used. Because not all sources of melatonin may have the same effect. SDPP application in the dry period has a positive effect on feed utilization as well as postpartum milk yield. In the studies, adding melatonin instead of applying SDPP in the dry period did not show the same effects. More studies are needed on the relationship between melatonin feeding and performance in dairy cattle. Milk yield parameters in sheep and goats depend on melatonin and prolactin concentrations as much as dairy cows. Using melatonin as a feed additive can reduce the stress caused by injection and implant applications. The use of exogenous melatonin as a subcutaneous implant together with naturally produced endogenous melatonin under SDPP conditions had no effect on lactation performances in different breeds of sheep with different levels of milk production level [29, 30]. This situation can be associated with the stress created in animals.

Rumen fermentation is an issue to be considered when using melatonin as a feed additive or oral preparation. Digestive enzymes and microorganisms in the rumen can metabolize melatonin. If melatonin is involved in rumen fermentation, its bioavailability may be significantly reduced. Therefore, melatonin should be tried in different forms (preserved or by-pass) and by adding it to the rations at different levels. Because it has been reported that the protein, fat and dry matter of milk increased in cows given melatonin in rumen protected from [31]. These researchers also emphasized that milk lactose level decreased with the addition of melatonin. The effect of preserved melatonin on nutrient digestibility or nutrient availability of cows should be considered as reasons for these results. Melatonin is an environmentally friendly molecule that is not toxic in the organism and its preserved forms are quite useful. For the treatment of mastitis, it may be recommended to use protected form of melatonin instead of antibiotics. Thus, the treatment cost would decrease, and the milk quality would increase. It has been determined that melatonin has an effect on some carcass parameters in beef cattle. In heifers given melatonin (4 mg/100 kg body weight) daily for 59 days, rib and longissimus muscle adiposity increased, carcass protein deposition decreased, but body weight gain was not affected [32].

5. The importance of melatonin hormone in laying hens and broiler chickens

The cycle of light and dark, which lasts for about 24 h, causes cyclical changes in birds. These cyclical, physiological, biochemical and behavioral effects are defined as circadian rhythm. The circadian rhythm in birds is highly synchronized by the pineal gland, retina and hypothalamus. Melatonin, the major hormone of the pineal gland, plays a role in controlling circadian rhythms in poultry [33].

Light intensity and duration of lighting also play an important role in the secretion of hormones that play a role in growth, maturation, reproduction and circadian rhythm in poultry. Circadian rhythms are important biological features of broilers and laying hens and are synchronized by daylight. The melatonin hormone secreted from the pineal gland plays a major role in this synchronization. The secretion of melatonin from the pineal gland in the dark is a reflection of this biological clock [34].

Broilers cannot achieve daily synchronization without melatonin. Most of the melatonin in the bloodstream is secreted in the pineal gland, but a small amount of melatonin is also produced in the enterochromaffin cells of the small intestinal mucosa. Melatonin production in the gastrointestinal tract is particularly associated with the consumption of diets rich in tryptophan. Because tryptophan is a structural component of protein and a precursor of the hormones serotonin and melatonin, which play an important role in maintaining normal physiological processes in broilers such as tissue regeneration, feed consumption, growth performance, feed conversion ratio and immunity [35]. The highest serum melatonin level occurs at midnight and is lowest at noon. However, the secretion of this hormone by mucosal enteroendocrine cells is associated with feed consumption and feeding frequency rather than photoperiod [36]. Orally administered melatonin to monogastric animals has high intestinal absorption and high bioavailability.

Another important role of melatonin in the organism is to participate in the antioxidant system and to protect cells from the harmful effects of free radicals. Inadequate secretion of melatonin in broilers causes metabolic and physiological disorders leading to reproductive diseases and deaths, thus economic losses [37]. Drugs and other methods used for the treatment of metabolic diseases are expensive and can negatively affect efficiency. Public health may also be adversely affected by the use of drugs in poultry. For this reason, it is important to use feed additives such as melatonin, which have no side effects, in order to prevent metabolic diseases that may occur. Apart from its use as a feed additive, melatonin is found in different parts of various plants. Oats and sweet corn take the first place with their melatonin content. In addition, walnuts, tomatoes, grapes, hazelnuts, strawberries, cherries and sour cherries contain significant amounts of melatonin [38]. It is thought that feeds rich in melatonin will positively affect the metabolic and physiological functions of birds. Thus, animal welfare problems caused by intense and long-term lighting can be compensated in this way.

5.1 Effects of melatonin supplementation on performance and health in laying hens and broilers

High productivity, rapid growth and intensive metabolism of broilers and layer hens are accompanied by excessive free radical formation. In addition, intense and prolonged light exposure may increase the risk of ascites and sudden death syndrome by preventing melatonin production [39]. Implementation of intermitted lighting programs in broiler farming resulted in decreased death rate and foot problems. Such lighting programs provide the opportunity to rest, less stress and high melatonin synthesis during the dark period [40]. Relić et al. added 30 mg/kg synthetic melatonin to broiler rations by applying continuous lighting for the first 2 weeks. At the end of the study, higher body weight gain in the group added melatonin to the feed was determined [35] . In another study where laying hens were supplemented with 10, 20 and

30 mg melatonin per animal, it was reported that the optimal dose for the best egg production and quality was 10 mg. At the same time, positive effects of melatonin on egg weight, shell thickness, albumin height and haugh unit parameters were reported. The rate of ovulation also shows a positive correlation with the level of melatonin in the blood, but the use of 30 mg negatively affected egg production and quality [41].

Although it has been stated that melatonin and its metabolites promote follicle maturation and ovulation by scavenging free radicals [42], high-dose melatonin supplementation may compromise the beneficial effect on ovulation by suppressing the physiological function of the ovaries. In order to evaluate the controversial results on this subject more meaningfully, the effects of different doses of melatonin on ovarian functions should be revealed in future studies. In a study examining melatonin effects on growth and development revealed that femur and tibia bones of chickens supplemented with melatonin were stronger. However, it caused a decrease in egg shell resistance [43]. The bone-strengthening effects of melatonin supplementation in chickens may be beneficial for poultry, but poor eggshell is undesirable. Therefore, melatonin supplementation may be more appropriate for broilers rather than layers. Although it has positive effects on laying hens, the melatonin metabolism of these animals is not known exactly.

Melatonin has effects on energy metabolism of broilers. In a study, physical activity decreased in animals placed in chambers for 20 days and exposed to intermittent lighting (16 h light-8 h dark) and added 40 ppm melatonin to their feed, thus energy loss was reduced. This effect was not observed in animals that exposed continuous lighting (23 h light-1 h dark) [6]. It is expected that the conserved energy that spent for physical activity positively affect the rate of feed conversion in broilers. Normally broilers do not eat at night. If they are exposed to continuous lighting, their feed consumption is considered to reach their maximum. However, several studies have shown that intermittent lighting programs improve body weight gain and feed efficiency, as well as reduce leg problems and mortality in broilers [44, 45]. The immune system strengthening effect of the increased melatonin secretion during the dark period helps to lower the mortality rate in poultry. In addition, application of melatonin alleviates the harmful effects of continuous lighting on broilers.

Melatonin plays a role in the development and maturation of the immune system. Stimulation of cytokine production, which increases lymphocyte activity, is one of its effects on immunity. Melatonin also increases the lethal activity of T cells and the production of interleukin and interferon in monocytes [46]. Melatonin hormone is also effective in regeneration of intestinal cells in poultry [36]. In a histopathological study, it was revealed that lymphoid hyperplasia in the liver, spleen and bursa fabricus was induced in broiler chickens treated with the addition of melatonin to the diet [47]. This result can be explained by the immunostimulating effect of melatonin. Bursa fabricus, which is involved in lymphocyte production in chickens, is suggested to be the target organ of melatonin [48]. It has been reported that 10–40 mg/kg melatonin supplementation significantly alleviates hepatic degeneration, necrosis and biliary hyperplasia resulting from aflatoxin in chicks [49]. This hormone may also interact with the thermoregulation mechanism in poultry. It has been reported that the body temperature of the 14-21d old and 150 mg/kg melatonin supplemented broiler chicks decreased and the heat distribution was regulated [50]. Melatonin can prolong life span by protecting erythrocytes in the blood from oxidative stress. It also stimulates the production of immune system cells such as lymphocytes, monocytes and eosinophils [51]. However, in another study, melatonin supplementation in broiler diets did not make a significant difference on hematological parameters [35].

Tryptophan, a precursor of melatonin, was used as an additive, increased cellular and humoral immunity, stimulated melatonin synthesis, and increased immunity by peritoneal macrophages reported as a result of the immunomodulatory effect of melatonin [52]. The effect of tryptophan on immune function is mediated by melatonin receptors in tissues. Patil et al. showed that tryptophan is a precursor of melatonin and inhibits oxidative damage in broilers, and also improves the enzymatic effect of catalase and superoxide dismutase [53]. However, Wang et al. emphasized that 1.5 times increased tryptophan level in the diet of broiler chickens housed under stress conditions, feed efficiency increased and oxidative stress reduced [54].

The optimal lighting level and the most appropriate feeding method are still being discussed in the poultry industry, where it is expected to achieve high level yield and production. With this expectation, animals are faced with stress factors such as intensive feeding and poultry housing conditions. Considering the properties of reducing stress factors, antioxidant and positive effects on animal health, the use of melatonin as an additive in poultry has been approved in many studies [35, 52].

6. Conclusions and recommendations

Feed additives are frequently studied and new products are introduced to the market in order to keep the function animal metabolism healthy. A wide variety of additives are used in order to protect animal health at the maximum level, to obtain higher efficiency and direct animal products according to consumer and market demands. Melatonin has positive effects, especially on the productivity of poultry. However, different melatonin sources should be tested on animals in different life periods. The effects of melatonin, which is used as a feed additive and as an implant, on ruminant animals are not certain. As a result of a small number of studies in ruminant animals, it has been found that only daylight and lighting duration are sometimes more effective than melatonin feeding. Apart from melatonin secreted by animals at night, the effects of melatonin added to feed should be examined in more detailed studies. The effects of melatonin as a silage additive, should be investigated on the most commonly ensiling forages used in ruminant feeding. Benefits of melatonin on silage quality by comparing it with other additives that affect silage fermentation should be proven. In conclusion, melatonin is a promising feed additive whose antioxidant and immune system support properties have been proven in many studies in animals.

Author details

Oğuzhan Kahraman, Zekeriya Safa İnanç*, Huzur Derya Arık
and Mustafa Selçuk Alataş
Faculty of Veterinary Medicine, Department of Animal Nutrition and Nutritional Diseases, Selcuk University, Konya, Turkey

*Address all correspondence to: zsafa.inanc@selcuk.edu.tr

References

[1] Li J, Liu J, Zhu T, Zhao C, Li L, Chen M. The role of melatonin in salt stress responses. International Journal of Molecular Sciences. 2019;**20**(7):1735. DOI: 10.3390/ijms20071735

[2] Pardo-Hernández M, López-Delacalle M, Rivero RM. ROS and NO regulation by melatonin under abiotic stress in plants. Antioxidants. 2020;**9**(11):1078. DOI: 10.20944/preprints202010.0051.v1

[3] Nawaz MA, Huang Y, Bie Z, Ahmed W, Reiter RJ, Niu M, et al. Melatonin: Current status and future perspectives in plant science. Frontiers in Plant Science. 2016;**6**:1230. DOI: 10.3389/fpls.2015.01230

[4] Pang S, Pang C, Poon A, Wan Q, Song Y, Brown G. An overview of melatonin and melatonin receptors in birds. Poultry and Avian Biology Reviews (United Kingdom). 1996;**7**(4):217-228

[5] Bermudez F, Forbes J, Injidi M. Involvement of melatonin and thyroid hormones in the control of sleep, food intake and energy metabolism in the domestic fowl. The Journal of Physiology. 1983;**337**(1):19-27. DOI: 10.1113/jphysiol.1983.sp014608

[6] Apeldoorn E, Schrama J, Mashaly M, Parmentier H. Effect of melatonin and lighting schedule on energy metabolism in broiler chickens. Poultry Science. 1999;**78**(2):223-229. DOI: 10.1093/ps/78.2.223

[7] Lerner AB, Case JD, Takahashi Y, Lee TH, Mori W. Isolation of melatonin, the pineal gland factor that lightens melanocyteS1. Journal of the American Chemical Society. 1958;**80**(10):2587. DOI: 10.1021/ja01543a060

[8] Reiter RJ. The melatonin rhythm: Both a clock and a calendar. Experientia. 1993;**49**(8):654-664. DOI: 10.1007/BF01923947

[9] Hardeland R, Poeggeler B. Non-vertebrate melatonin. Journal of Pineal Research. 2003;**34**(4):233-241. DOI: 10.1034/j.1600-079x.2003.00040.x

[10] Skaper S, Floreani M, Ceccon M, Facci L, Giusti P. Excitotoxicity, oxidative stress, and the neuroprotective potential of melatonin. Annals of the New York Academy of Sciences. 1999;**890**(1):107-118. DOI: 10.1111/j.1749-6632.1999.tb07985.x

[11] Valko M, Leibfritz D, Moncol J, Cronin MT, Mazur M, Telser J. Free radicals and antioxidants in normal physiological functions and human disease. The International Journal of Biochemistry & Cell Biology. 2007;**39**(1):44-84. DOI: 10.1016/j.biocel.2006.07.001

[12] Vanecek J. Cellular mechanisms of melatonin action. Physiological Reviews. 1998;**78**(3):687-721. DOI: 10.1152/physrev.1998.78.3.687

[13] Reiter RJ. Cytoprotective properties of melatonin: Presumed association with oxidative damage and aging. Nutrition. 1998;**14**(9):691-696. DOI: 10.1016/s0899-9007(98)00064-1

[14] Watson RR. Melatonin in the Promotion of Health. CRC Press; 2011

[15] Dominguez-Rodriguez A, Abreu-Gonzalez P, Avanzas P. The role of melatonin in acute myocardial infarction. Frontiers in Bioscience. 2012;**17**:2433-2441. DOI: 10.2741/4063

[16] Nabavi SM, Nabavi SF, Sureda A, Xiao J, Dehpour AR, Shirooie S, et al. Anti-inflammatory effects of melatonin: A mechanistic review. Critical Reviews in Food Science and Nutrition. 2019;**59**(supl):S4-S16. DOI: 10.1080/10408398.2018.1487927

[17] Khripach V, Zhabinskii V, de Groot A. Twenty years of brassinosteroids: Steroidal plant hormones warrant better crops for the XXI century. Annals of Botany. 2000;**86**(3):441-447. DOI: 10.1006/anbo.2000.1227

[18] Bashir T, Naz S, Bano A. Plant growth promoting rhizobacteria in combination with plant growth regulators attenuate the effect of drought stress. Pakistan Journal of Botany. 2020;**52**(3):783-792. DOI: 10.30848/PJB2020-3(17)

[19] Byeon Y, Back K. Melatonin synthesis in rice seedlings in vivo is enhanced at high temperatures and under dark conditions due to increased serotonin N-acetyltransferase and N-acetylserotonin methyltransferase activities. Journal of Pineal Research. 2014;**56**(2):189-195. DOI: 10.1111/jpi.12111

[20] Hasan MK, Ahammed GJ, Yin L, Shi K, Xia X, Zhou Y, et al. Melatonin mitigates cadmium phytotoxicity through modulation of phytochelatins biosynthesis, vacuolar sequestration, and antioxidant potential in *Solanum lycopersicum* L. Frontiers in Plant Science. 2015;**6**:601. DOI: 10.3389/fpls.2015.00601

[21] Azizi F, Amiri H, Ismaili A. Melatonin improves salinity stress tolerance of *Phaseolus vulgaris* L. cv. Pak by changing antioxidant enzymes and photosynthetic parameters. Acta Physiologiae Plantarum. 2022;**44**(4):1-12. DOI: 0.1007/s11738-022-03373-y

[22] Muck R, Nadeau E, McAllister T, Contreras-Govea F, Santos M, Kung L Jr. Silage review: Recent advances and future uses of silage additives. Journal of Dairy Science. 2018;**101**(5):3980-4000. DOI: 10.3168/jds.2017-13839

[23] Li M, Lv R, Zhang L, Zi X, Zhou H, Tang J. Melatonin is a promising silage additive: Evidence from microbiota and metabolites. Frontiers in Microbiology. 2021;**12**:670764. DOI: 10.3389/fmicb.2021.670764

[24] Ponchon B, Lacasse P, Ollier S, Zhao X. Effects of photoperiod modulation and melatonin feeding around drying-off on bovine mammary gland involution. Journal of Dairy Science. 2017;**100**(10):8496-8506. DOI: 10.3168/jds.2016-12272

[25] Sanchez-Barcelo E, Mediavilla M, Zinn S, Buchanan B, Chapin L, Allen TH. Melatonin suppression of mammary growth in heifers. Biology of Reproduction. 1991;**44**(5):875-879

[26] Dahl G, Buchanan B, Tucker H. Photoperiodic effects on dairy cattle: A review. Journal of Dairy Science. 2000;**83**(4):885-893. DOI: 10.1095/biolreprod44.5.875

[27] Garcia-Ispierto I, Abdelfatah A, López-Gatius F. Melatonin treatment at dry-off improves reproductive performance postpartum in high-producing dairy cows under heat stress conditions. Reproduction in Domestic Animals. 2013;**48**(4):577-583. DOI: 10.1111/rda.12128

[28] Lanoix D, Lacasse A-A, Reiter RJ, Vaillancourt C. Melatonin: The watchdog of villous trophoblast homeostasis against hypoxia/reoxygenation-induced oxidative stress and apoptosis. Molecular and Cellular Endocrinology. 2013;**381**(1-2):35-45. DOI: 10.1016/j.mce.2013.07.010

[29] Cosso G, Mura MC, Pulinas L, Curone G, Vigo D, Carcangiu V, et al. Effects of melatonin treatment on milk traits, reproductive performance and immune response in Sarda dairy sheep. Italian Journal of Animal Science. 2021;**20**(1):632-639. DOI: 10.1080/1828051X.2021.1904796

[30] Elhadi A, Salama A, Such X, Caja G. Responses to melatonin of 2 breeds of dairy ewes in early lactation under autumn photoperiod conditions. Journal of Dairy Science. 2022;**105**(3):2587-2596. DOI: 10.3168/jds.2021-21270

[31] Yao S, Wu H, Ma H, Fu Y, Wei W, Wang T, et al. Effects of rumen bypass melatonin feeding (RBMF) on milk quality and mastitis of Holstein cows. PeerJ. 2020;**8**:e9147. DOI: 10.7717/peerj.9147

[32] Zinn S, Chapin L, Enright W, Schroeder A, Stanisiewski E, Tucker H. Growth, carcass composition and plasma melatonin in postpubertal beef heifers fed melatonin. Journal of Animal Science. 1988;**66**(1):21-27. DOI: 10.2527/jas1988.66121x

[33] Hieke A-SC, Hubert SM, Athrey G. Circadian disruption and divergent microbiota acquisition under extended photoperiod regimens in chicken. PeerJ. 2019;**7**:e6592. DOI: 10.7717/peerj.6592

[34] Trivedi AK, Kumar V. Melatonin: An internal signal for daily and seasonal timing. 2014;**52**(5):425-437

[35] Relić R, Škrbić Z, Božičković I, Lukić M, Petričević V, Delić N, et al. Effects of dietary melatonin on broiler chicken exposed to continuous lighting during the first two weeks of life. Ankara Üniversitesi Veteriner Fakültesi Dergisi. 2022. DOI: 10.33988/auvfd.866702. Available from: http://vetjournal.ankara.edu.tr/tr/pub/issue/48904

[36] Liu L, Zhang S, Bao J, He X, Tong D, Chen C, et al. Melatonin improves laying performance by enhancing intestinal amino acids transport in hens. Frontiers in Endocrinology. 2018;**9**:426. DOI: 10.3389/fendo.2018.00426

[37] Zhao D, Yu Y, Shen Y, Liu Q, Zhao Z, Sharma R, et al. Melatonin synthesis and function: Evolutionary history in animals and plants. Frontiers in Endocrinology. 2019;**10**:249. DOI: 10.3389/fendo.2019.00249

[38] Calislar S, Yeter B, Sahin A. Importance of melatonin on poultry. 2018;**21**(6):987-997. DOI: 10.18016/ksutarimdoga.vi.433039

[39] Underwood H, Goldman BD. Vertebrate circadian and photoperiodic systems: Role of the pineal gland and melatonin. Journal of Biological Rhythms. 1987;**2**(4):279-315. DOI: 10.1177/074873048700200404

[40] Başer E, Yetişir R. Farklı aydınlatma programlarının etlik piliç performansı ve refahı üzerine etkisi. Hayvansal Üretim. 2010;**51**(2):68-76

[41] Jia Y, Yang M, Zhu K, Wang L, Song Y, Wang J, et al. Melatonin implantation improved the egg-laying rate and quality in hens past their peak egg-laying age. Scientific Reports. 2016;**6**(1):1-8. DOI: 10.1038/srep39799

[42] Galano A, Tan DX, Reiter RJ. Melatonin as a natural ally against oxidative stress: A physicochemical examination. Journal of Pineal Research. 2011;**51**(1):1-16. DOI: 10.1111/j.1600-079X.2011.00916.x

[43] Taylor AC, Horvat-Gordon M, Moore A, Bartell PA. The effects of melatonin on the physical properties of bones and egg shells in the laying hen.

PLoS One. 2013;**8**(2):e55663. DOI: 10.1371/journal.pone.0055663

[44] Buyse J, Decuypere E, Michels H. Intermittent lighting and broiler production. 1. Effect on female broiler performance. Archiv für Geflügelkunde. 1994;**58**(2):69

[45] Yang H, Xing H, Wang Z, Xia J, Wan Y, Hou B, et al. Effects of intermittent lighting on broiler growth performance, slaughter performance, serum biochemical parameters and tibia parameters. Italian Journal of Animal Science. 2015;**14**(4):4143. DOI: 10.4081/ijas.2015.4143

[46] Skwarlo-Sonta K. Melatonin in immunity: Comparative aspects. Neuroendocrinology Letters. 2002;**23**:61-66

[47] Ahmed HH, Essawy GS, Salem HA, Abd el-daim MA. Effect of melatonin on some hematological parameters and immune status of broiler chicks. Journal of Agricultural Science. 2011;**3**(2):243. DOI: 10.1016/j.cca.2003.10.008

[48] Lee PP, Pang SF. Identification and characterization of melatonin binding sites in the gastrointestinal tract of ducks. Life Sciences. 1992;**50**(2):117-125. DOI: 10.1016/0024-3205(92)90293-x

[49] Özen H, Karaman M, Çiğremiş Y, Tuzcu M, Özcan K, Erdağ D. Effectiveness of melatonin on aflatoxicosis in chicks. Research in Veterinary Science. 2009;**86**(3):485-489. DOI: 10.1016/j.rvsc.2008.09.011

[50] Zeman M, Buyse J, Herichova I, Decuypere E. Melatonin decreases heat production in female broiler chickens. Acta Veterinaria Brno. 2001;**70**(1):15-18. DOI: 10.1093/ps/78.2.223

[51] Calvo JR, Gonzalez-Yanes C, Maldonado M. The role of melatonin in the cells of the innate immunity: A review. Journal of Pineal Research. 2013;**55**(2):103-120. DOI: 10.1111/jpi.12075

[52] Mund MD, Riaz M, Mirza MA, Rahman Z, Mahmood T, Ahmad F, et al. Effect of dietary tryptophan supplementation on growth performance, immune response and anti-oxidant status of broiler chickens from 7 to 21 days. Veterinary Medicine and Science. 2020;**6**(1):48-53. DOI: 10.1002/vms3.195

[53] Patil R, Tyagi J, Sirajudeen M, Singh R, Moudgal R, Mohan J. Effect of dietary melatonin and L-tryptophan on growth performance and immune responses of broiler chicken under experimental aflatoxicosis. Iranian Journal of Applied Animal Science. 2013;**3**(1):139-144

[54] Wang B, Min Z, Yuan J, Zhang B, Guo Y. Effects of dietary tryptophan and stocking density on the performance, meat quality, and metabolic status of broilers. Journal of Animal Science and Biotechnology. 2014;**5**(1):1-7. DOI: 10.1186/2049-1891-5-44